Dedicatio

This book is dedicated to the students, alumni and staff of Freeman Schools. There is something to be said about being Freeman Strong. There's a grittiness that exists there. Maybe it is in the dirt, maybe it is in the hearts of the farmers who live there. I know I have a lot to be thankful for when it comes to growing up Freeman Strong. If it wasn't for my Freeman education I wouldn't have had the tools I needed to cure my disease. Although they recently suffered a terrifying and life-changing school shooting, I know that the heart of Freeman still beats. I was lucky enough to have been spared the terror that is school shootings. I do not know why. I certainly did not deserve to be spared. Honestly, I didn't deserve even a scratch of pen from them and still they taught me. They gave me an education and they taught me to never give up. That is why I know they will come out of this stronger. Even more Freeman Strong than ever before.

My Diagnosis

I always thought I was more prone to the stomach flu than others. I spent decades with this disease, not really understanding I had a condition and wasn't just more susceptible to the stomach flu or food poisoning.

There is no cure for this disease and no definitive cause. Although it is being studied.

Often children who suffer from migraines will come down with this disease. About three out of every 100,000 children will come down with cyclic vomiting syndrome or what some refer to as abdominal migraines.

Females are slightly more prone to get this disease and while all races have been afflicted, it does seem to affect Caucasians the most.

Some studies say that chronic marijuana use can cause the symptoms associated with cyclic vomiting syndrome. While the symptoms are very similar, chronic marijuana use can cause a condition known as cannabinoid hyperemesis. A suffer such as myself, who has spent years being a frequent visitor to the Emergency Room, can tell you that this comparison is something I'm fairly sensitive about. This disease is just now getting recognized by the public and by the medical community. Before, when I went into the emergency room I would at first be labeled as what medical professionals refer to as a drug seeker. A drug seeker is someone who goes to the emergency room with the intention of tricking doctors into prescribing pain medications and who doesn't necessarily suffer from a medical condition. Because I was always initially screened as a drug seeker, it's fairly important to me that I don't use or be associated with marijuana or any other street drugs. There's a lot of information about that differentiates between cannabis hyperemis and my condition of cyclic vomiting syndrome.

Dysfunctional mitochondria has been suggested as a cause of the disease. The mitochondria are located in every cell of the body but the red blood cells. Because the mitochondria play a large role in energy production in the body, I refer to them as the car battery and our bodies the car. In order to get the car (the human body) to properly turn over, the battery needs to be fully charged.

Mitochondrial disease is its own illness. Symptoms of this disease include poor growth, loss of muscle coordination, muscle weakness, visual problems, hearing problems, learning disabilities, heart disease, liver disease, kidney disease, gastrointestinal disorders, respiratory disorders, neurological problems, autonomic dysfunction and dementia. Currently there is no cure for mitochondrial disease although there is a test for it. There is no test for cyclical vomiting syndrome.

Though there are no current medications for cyclic vomiting syndrome, enzymes like Co-Q10 and L-Carnitine that both aide in the ATP energy production in the cells has been used with success. Other migraine medications such as Sumatriptan have shown to ease the severity of the symptoms. There has even been a recent development of nasal Sumatriptan to aide patients experiencing an episode.

Often when I would visit an emergency room, most medical professionals had never experienced a symptomatic cyclical vomiting syndrome patient. Most people probably wouldn't necessarily understand why a patient experiencing a CVS episode would need IV. medications such as Zofran or Reglan, or even intravenous fluids. When a person is having a cyclical vomiting episode they simply cannot stop vomiting. They vomit to the point of severe dehydration from fluid loss. In order to recoup fluids the vomiting must stop and/or fluids must be given to the patient. Occasionally if I managed to get to the hospital before I reached the point of dehydration, I would be given an injection to stop the vomiting. Usually though, I would go to the emergency room already dehydrated, need IV. fluids, and given a cocktail of drugs to try and stop the vomiting. It usually took hours, but so far the vomiting episodes have always ceased. When I am having an episode I vomit approximately six times per hour. I would come down with an episode about 3-4 times per year. Now that I'm on enzyme therapy (CO-Q10, L-Carnitine, Creatine) and exercise treatment, I've only had one episode in the last three years.

When I'm not symptomatic, other than recovering being bedridden for days, my life is fairly normal. That's why this disease is referred to as an invisible illness. It's so invisible I didn't even see any huge difference between myself and other healthy individuals. Perhaps I also suffered from optimism bias in that I wanted to be a healthy happy individual so much, I simply refused to see that my body wasn't like everyone else's. However, I see it now. I'm doing something about it. I've never felt more healthy or been happier.

I remember when I finally got to a gastroenterologist and was diagnosed officially with cyclic vomiting syndrome. My doctor told me there was no cure and really nothing he could do to help me. Honestly, that diagnosis was all I needed. I heard the words and I was off!

I'm still reeling in happiness knowing that I have a condition and not a weakened immune system. I was able to learn how to control my symptoms, although I will likely always be chronically ill. I've learned how to live with my chronic illness. I've learned how to manage my symptoms and how to live better with chronic illness. It really is an answered prayer. For years I lived from goal-to-goal as I thought I didn't have much of a future full of wellness. I see a future now. I have dreams now. I never had those. Dreams are gifts from God. I am so thankful everyday that I get to see a future ahead of me now that's not full of Emergency Room visits and saline tubes. That's why I wrote this book. I want to help you help yourself. I want to help you learn how to live better with chronic illness.

Sources

https://en.wikipedia.org/wiki/Mitochondrial_disease

http://www.niddk.nih.gov/health-information/health-topics/digestive-diseases/cyclic-vomiting-syndrome/Pages/facts.aspx

http://www.mayoclinic.org/diseases-conditions/cyclic-vomiting-syndrome/basics/definition/con-20028160

https://en.wikipedia.org/wiki/Cyclic_vomiting_syndrome

http://www.hightimes.com/read/what-cannabinoid-hyperemesis-syndrome

http://nursinglink.monster.com/benefits/articles/9065-top-10-signs-your-patient-may-be-a-drug-seeker

My Religion

Yes, I am a Seventh Day Adventist. I attended Seventh Day Adventist bible camp. Seventh Day Adventists are considered to be among the blue zone group. The term blue zone refers to the characteristics of a group of people who are known to live the longest in the world. Seventh Day Adventists live over a hundred years on a regular basis and a study in *National Geographic Magazine* showcased specific characteristics of people who live the longest in the world. One of those was the group of people who identify as Seventh Day Adventists. The easy answer to who these people are and who I am are Christians who worship on Saturdays and don't witness the way other Christians do.

This has been my biggest struggle. There have been so many times that I've felt like I was well beneath the standard living of a Seventh Day Adventist. I've been guilty of smoking cigarettes on occasion and I still drink wine. Oh, and I also eat bacon. I was raised under the guidance of this wonderful religion, but I fall short in so many categories. The one thing about the SDAs that I do carry with me is their belief in how you should witness to non-believers. I witness by example. I would never tell anyone they are wrong for what they believe. I wake up every morning and ask God to help me be a good person, to not lie and try and spread kindness. He answers my prayers most days – even with someone as unfortunate as me. The reason I am here is the other tenant of this religion that I carry deep inside me. That is good ol' American grit. Being an American born religion, us Seventh Day Adventists have been known to do all sorts of things that involves dirt and grime and come out of it unscathed. We ain't afraid of getting dirt under our nails. We get the job done. It is with this grittiness that I managed to abate the symptoms of my chronic illness.

When I was officially diagnosed and told there was no cure and nothing my doctor could do for me, I went to the books and started reading. I started researching and taking health classes. I wasn't giving up. I wasn't going to let this chronic illness be the death of me. I had CVS, but CVS didn't have me.

The first thing I did was change my diet. I then began exercising. I remember when I first hit the treadmill at the gym. I have never been much of an athlete. I put my sneakers on the belt and set my treadmill to a low pace and walked. I wasn't really too much of a runner. I looked at the person next to me. She was running at a way faster pace than me. I almost got off the treadmill at that point. I'd never stop my illness. It was destroying me. It would soon lick me. My body was compromised. I was this close to giving up and letting go.

But I didn't.

I stayed on the treadmill. I ignored the person running next to me and focused on my own steps. I never got very fast as a runner, but what I didn't know was that I was benefitting my mitochondria by engaging in aerobic exercise. Suh, huh?

Aerobic Vs. Anaerobic Exercise

If you are anything like me, and not someone who ever thought they would become an exercise junkie, then you may not know the difference between aerobic and anaerobic exercise.

Sometimes called cardio, aerobic exercise is physical exercise that starts low and goes to high intensity. It took me years to realize why I was so bad at aerobic exercise. In fact, I was regularly the slowest runner in my physical exercise class. It's a little known fact that aerobic exercise actually makes the mitochondria healthier. Let me caveat once again: I'm not a scientist. I'm a journalist with a high I.Q. When I began my journey to wellness I hit the books. I studied the health sciences. I did this because there were no answers to how to cure my illness. I have always been someone who has embraced western medicine. Had I had an option to take a pill, I would have done that. This was the only option I had. Had I not done what I did, I would have ended up carried by six and dumped in the ground.

The reason that aerobic exercise is so good for the body and the mitochondria is how it utilizes oxygen in the body to make energy. The definition of aerobic is "relating to, involving, or requiring free oxygen."

The cardio process involves breathing. As breathing becomes heavier the body is then forced to get to work. This process makes the body better. That's why exercise is such an important part of Living Better with Chronic Illness. We've all been bombarded with these mega-svelt people with abs of steel who are looking down on all of us and our jiggly spots. Well, they have their rent to pay to. For the rest of us, know that some aerobic exercise is better than none. If high intensity training is not your thing, start with a walk at the park. That's better than nothing and it still has health benefits.

Mitochondria, Huh What?

The scientific definition of mitochondrion is *An organelle found in large numbers in most cells, in which the biochemical processes of respiration and energy production occur.*

Now that's a mouthful. Basically, mitochondria are a part of every cell that makes up our amazing bodies. I refer to them as the battery and our bodies the car – fyi, I worked on a lot of cars in my youth. Now, our body's cells make up the energy that allows our bodies to perform. It then transfers the energy to the various parts of our bodies that make it function right. The mitochondria play an integral role in this production. Regular aerobic exercise improves the function of the mitochondria. If you're someone like me who has mitochondria that are a little weak, then that will impact the entire function of the body.

When I read this, I said to myself that I needed to pump up my mitochondria if I wanted to learn how to Live Better with Chronic Illness. That was the key to unlocking my inner strength. I needed to improve the function of my body's car battery if I wanted to stop going to the Emergency Room. So, I joined a gym. I hit the treadmill. I then gave up doughnuts. I added steak to my diet. Yes, steak. Oh and fat. I started to eat fat.

As I got better the weight was not coming up. Plus, I lacked an appetite. I started doing hefty workouts just to feel hungry. I ate hamburgers without the bun and drank chocolate milk post-workout. I could feel my body improving. My frequent flyer visits to the Emergency Room ceased. I was getting better. For the first time in my life I was learning what it was like to have a somewhat healthy body. It was amazing. I still cannot believe I was allowed to know what it was like to feel healthy.

This book is about how I healed my mitochondria. So I will be talking a lot about these little guys. They are more important than anyone realizes. Everyone has mitochondria. Us mammals do not have mitochondria in our red blood cells. They are everywhere else though.

Fun Fact! The word mitochondria comes from the Greek word for thread.

Hence, it is the thread that maintains our health in our bodies. It starts getting compromised then all sorts of yucky things happen to our bodies.

Take mine for example. For years I used to puke – a lot. The mitochondria wear several hats in the role they play in our body function.

My disease isn't the only one that's been linked to faulty mitochondria. There are a list of mitochondrial disorders and the mitochondria have been implicated in the cause of cardiac dysfunction, heart failure and even autism.

Autism is kind of a heart wrenching term for me. I've pondered if I was on the spectrum disorder chart for years. I've never been able to quite fit in and have a lot of the characteristics. Probably the weirdest thing about curing my chronic illness, is that when I healed my body a lot of my characteristics of autism left too. There's something about physical health and autism. I don't know what. I'm a journalist, not a scientist. All I know is that when I took charge of my health, my personality problems healed themselves too. There's a link. I know not what.

With the cardiac or heart stuff, did you know that Charles Darwin is thought to have had cyclic vomiting syndrome. Likely caused my mitochondrial dysfunction. He died from heart failure.

Damage to the mitochondria can cause so many diseases. Back to the autism, mitochondrial disorders have been linked to neurological disorders like autism. It's also been linked to diseases like diabetes. Mitochondria are little, but are a big deal – especially when it comes to health. Other mental disorders like schizophremia, bipolar disorder, dementia, Alzheimer's disease, Parkinson's disease, epilepsy, stroke, cardiovascular disease, chronic fatigue syndrome, retina issues and diabetes.

The decrease in the mitochondria's function in the body has also been linked to aging. If you're like me ever looked at a workout guru in awe at their age and youthful appearance, then know that it may be that they look so good because they have such healthy mitochondria. I targeted the health of my mitochondria when I wanted to feel better. I've never felt better or looked better. People say all the time I don't look my age. When I was in my twenties I looked way older than I do now. The proof is in the mitochondria pudding, I guess.

When I began my journey to wellness and targeted my mitochondria I remember when I finally got the courage to go to a fitness class. I was scared. I was about to be surrounded by people in way better shape than me. I remember the first day of my first spinning class. I was way behind with a way bigger behind than my peers. I thought then how I was in the negative when it came to health. It would take a lot of peddling to make up for the health deficit I'd been in in my youth. I had some work to do if I was going to make up for all the lost health time I had when I was in my twenties. I needed to get to work.

After having a baby, I could not get the weight off. I ended up losing about thirty pounds when I became a gym rat. My worst class was always step. I thought it was confusing and the cardio component was brutal on my lungs. I will never forget how my fitness instructor took the time to break down the steps in a way that I could understand. She is my Earthly health angel.

My Cyclic Vomiting Syndrome

Like most high school seniors, I had a big decision to make.
What would I study? I knew that I was going to college no matter
what. I had too many people tell me I was garbage who I needed
to prove wrong. A pretty non-judgmental person myself with well-
developed empathy skills, I can understand why they thought I
was garbage—and in way that they were right. My hair was
generally unwashed along with my body, my face was covered in
acne, and for much of my adolescence I had a 100 percent
overbite. On top of that, skipping school was an easy decision for
me and was usually a regular thing. By my junior year, I had
been tested and knew my I.Q. was well above average sitting at
around 130 and they couldn't find enough questions to properly
test my vocabulary and comprehension skills. One might think
that this would make me beloved my by school, but it didn't. On

top of my undesirable looks, I missed quite a bit of school. Some of it was indeed me skipping out to visit the mall, but usually it was because I was involved in a regular process where I'd spend up to two weeks puking 4-6 times per hour. I had/have a disease called cyclic vomiting syndrome that wouldn't be diagnosed until my early 30s. At the cusp of adulthood my teenage self decided that I simply couldn't handle another person's vomiting and instead of nursing I went into journalism (a decision I do not regret BTW!)

So now here I am, in my early 30s with a resume of photography, editorial skills, communication and journalism going back to school to study the health sciences. Deciding to do this–like my decision to study journalism—was not solely mine. My disease cyclic vomiting syndrome is very rare, has no testing, and no treatment. Still, in more than four years since my diagnosis I have been able to abate most of my symptoms using enzymes that have been tested to aide mitochondria. Even after three years of independent study—and success!—I'm still a novice, however. Because I procreated before I found out that my body was severely compromised there is no other job more important to me than to try and stay in this world full of murderers, liars, and abusers so I can be there to protect my child.

Since my diagnoses my day dreams full of puppies and warm kisses were replaced by finding a doctor. Not just any doctor, but one interested in the uniqueness of my case. And I think maybe my day dreams have finally come true. Instead of shaking his head and saying he couldn't help me like doctors before him, this medical professional sent me home with literature. Despite my illness, one thing is certain: I do have amazing reading and comprehension skills. Some may call it wisdom, I happen to think I'm still too young to be considered wise. I very much appreciate a medical professional who sees me as someone who will do whatever it takes to manage my health, if not for me, for my daughter.

In the article he gave me, most of the information was not anything I hadn't read before. I am on a regular enzyme treatment that includes CoQ10, L-Carnitine, and creatine—all enzymes that benefit the mitochondria and the ATP energy system. Here is a link to the complete article:http://www.townsendletter.com/June2015/mito0615.htmlAre GM Foods Harming the Mitochondria?

The most heart-sinking for me in this article was this sentence: *"The mitochondria are subjected to a number of modern-day insults, including toxins. Although there are many toxins that impair mitochondrial function, one of the most prevalent is glyphosate (used in Roundup). Because genetically modified (GM) foods are engineered to be resistant to glyphosate, they're slathered with this herbicide."*

As a journalist who abhors bias, reading the above sentence for the first time caused me to begin to shake uncontrollably in anger. I have strong beliefs in keeping the powerful accountable and I do NOT like bullies. At the same time that I'm trying to keep my outrage in check, waves of anger that there could be someone out there who compromised My Life and My Physiology outrages me. Still, I have to keep my journalistic wits about me and I have to honor the scientific process. I will be finding scientists researching this glyphosate. I will be thoroughly vetting their scientific process to be sure we don't have another famous failed study that somehow managed to instead show that this chemical is harmless. And I will be talking about my disease in hopes that I can help people learn to Live Better with Chronic Illness.

I May Have CVS, But CVS Doesn't Have Me

I've yet to meet someone who has been to the pearly gates as much as me. So many times have I laid helpless on a gurney and asked God to have mercy on my pain and take me to heaven. If I've learned anything about life it's that sometimes God doesn't answer all our prayers. Existence for me right now is simply amazing. Had he answered those pitiful prayers that came from pain, I would never be here experiencing what I am experiencing right now. I feel the health of my body and I want to scream out in pure joy. Life is a gift and it is amazing. I also know that pain is awful and when I was sick I did not consider life to be a gift. I thought it was a horrible curse. I now know I was wrong. Thank goodness I was wrong.

Because of my Frequent Flyer status of the Emergency Room, I have certain habits that I cannot break. One is my underwear. Yes, I'm about to tell you about my underwear. I'm very cautious that it looks is best. I do my best with my outer garments as well.

There was little I could do for years about my frazzled appearance. I could do something about my clothes. I became a sickly fashionista. I bet my doctors were really impressed when they ordered the nurses to hold my puke bucket. I just talked about puking and panties in the same paragraph. Sauscum!

The thing about my cyclical vomiting syndrome and my response to it, is that I don't remember not having this disease. I have had extreme bouts of vomiting since I was a child. I missed a lot of school because of this strange disease. Frequently, I get people who like to criticize my mother for taking care of me at home instead of taking me to the emergency room. My response is always that if she had done that, then it wouldn't have changed anything. When I was sick my disease was unheard of. Plus, my mother was a very smart and talented nurse and I had the best care a person could ask for. Nowadays if a person pukes for more than two days they should go to the Emergency Room. Way back when I was a kid, you didn't do that. I would puke for weeks and not go to the doctor. But I was being taken care of.

It took a lot for me to go to the Emergency Room for the first time. I remember when I got there and was escorted to one of the hospital beds. I only had been vomiting for 24 hours, and they inserted an intravenous line into my veins and started a saline drip. I was feeling rehydrated. I really cannot properly describe the amazing feeling that comes from being on the brink of death to feeling your veins fill with fluid and become better. My only comparison is that of a dried out sponge, completely useless. It only becomes useful when you run it under the faucet and it absorbs water. I was that sponge. I hated being completely helpless and that saline drip brought me back from the brink of death. Another reason I am so thankful for existence.

People ask me all the time now how I can be such a health nut about food. I tell them that it sure beats a saline drip. I am so thankful for this technology, however, if I can avoid it I will. If that means eating fruits and veggies and taking enzymes, then I will. Now, in my diet I avoid wheat and legumes like lentils. I will say this repeatedly: I am not a gluten hater. I have an allergy. I feel this needs to be said. I'm not on a diet, I have a lifestyle. I have to live a healthy lifestyle in order to stay out of the Emergency Room. For some reason wheat triggers my illness as do lentils. Maybe it's the glyphosate, I do not know. What I do is that if I eat those foods I get sick. One thing else I know is that I am a farm girl. I was raised around wheat and lentil production. This seems like too much of a coincidence, but my journalism brain will not let me confirm the link until a scientist backs up this connection. I do know that the foods I'm allergic to, happen to be the foods that I was most around as a child. I can say that for sure.

I say that I may have cyclical vomiting syndrome but it doesn't have me, because I think life is a precious gift. Sure, there a billions of humans on the planet, but there is only one of you. It is up to you to live a good life. It is up to you to live a healthy life. If you eat too much you will face health problems. If you drink too much you will face health problems. I can't control that I have cyclical vomiting syndrome, I can control my reaction to it however. I choose to fight it. I know I will ultimately loose the battle. My disease is rare and very debilitating. I want to live. I want to live healthy. I will fight the symptoms of this disease as long as I can. If you choose to live a sedentary lifestyle, then it is your fault the scale keeps going up. There are loads of ways to get active and if you don't want six pack abs you don't have to have those. Your wellness does involve you however. I can only help you on your journey to wellness. You have to take the first step to Living better with Chronic Illness. It is up to you. Personally, I think you can do it. If someone has compromised as me could do it, certainly you can.

Coping With Chronic Illness When Everything Goes Down in Flames

The Yale Road Fire and the Community of Farmers That Saved a Town

I stood on a gravel road facing a ravine leading to majestic Valleyford's California Creek. Behind the southside of the steep drop off lay my property and behind that a giant plume of smoke. My cellphone rang. On the other end a friend called to ask if I was OK and had heard there was a fire out there. My words jumbled into the phone. The garbling sounds that came out of my mouth made no sense. On either side of me listening to my insane jargon, stood my neighbors who I rarely see who were probably thinking, "Tammy's at a loss for words? Wow, things must really be bad."

I finally managed to say, "This is really bad. This isn't good. No, I'm not OK."

Less than an hour prior my husband, 5-year-old daughter and I were traveling back from Rathdrum to rehome a cat that had belonged to his father who passed away the week before. The city of Rathdrum, ID sits a little over 30 miles northeast of the tiny town of Valleyford. The quaint town stretches across 12 miles of mostly farmland and hosts a little over 1,000 residents of mostly farmers, small producers, and country folk. For reference sake, let me say that I stand with one foot on either side of small producer and weird country bumpkin.

Valleyford sits just southeast of Spokane, Wash. and just south of Spokane Valley, Wash. about 10 miles.

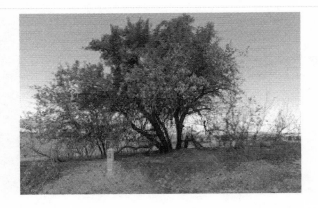

This apple tree that sits just north of Stoughton shows where the fire jumped the road and had it not been for diligent farmers and firefighters could have moved north and destroyed several homes.

Driving back from Rathdrum, I could see my husband still wore that deep sad look that can only come from a combination of grief, shock, and a still-recent painful event.

I squeezed his hand to signal that I was there for him. My cell phone rang. It was my neighbor. "Tammy, are you home?"

"No, we haven't been home all week. We've been dealing with my father-in-law's death. We had a funeral to plan and estate to settle."

"Tammy there's a fire. It's headed our way. I'm not evacuating yet, but I'm in my car ready to go."

I hung up the phone and looked out the driver's window. I could see a plume of smoke in the horizon southwest of me.

"This couldn't be headed towards my house? My husband's dad just died. My luck couldn't be that bad," I thought.

When we pulled into my driveway, we could see the cloud of smoke blanket the sky. My surroundings grew dark and looked like evening time although it wasn't even 4 p.m. My husband let us out then hopped back into the car, "I want to go see where the fire is," he said then abruptly left.

I nodded then proceeded to follow my usual routine of going inside to let the dogs out while my 5-year-old investigated for eggs in the chicken coop.

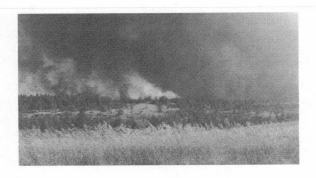

My view from the ravine where we evacuated.

The sky became darker and the cloud of smoke grew larger. A mixture of shock between the recent loss of a family member and this current crisis, I followed my routine. I let my dogs out and went out into the backyard to check my garden for any newly ripened vegetables.

Finally though, the sound of fire shook me out of my calm confused state.

I come from a long line of strong women. Some were logger wives, farm wives, or like me the daughter of a hard-as-nails nurse who spent 40 years serving sick people at Sacred Heart

Medical Center in Spokane. I wouldn't know how to wring my hands and bawl if someone showed me.

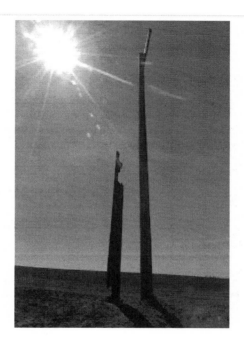

Whether this pole was replaced after the windstorm in 2015 or the recent fire, it does show how destructive fire can be.

The week prior, when I got the call that my father-in-law was at the CICU or Cardiac Intensive Care Unit I hung up and jumped in my vehicle and headed straight to the hospital that has been such an important part of my life. Born there, fed there, raised by one of the employees of this facility; I knew I was about to see someone take their last breath there. The last text read that they had performed CPR on my father-in-law for the third time. The daughter of a nurse and a professional rescuer myself, I knew things were not looking good.

Sitting across from my husband in the waiting room that only an hour before held a dozen or more people praying for a miracle, the news came that he was gone and I could see the look of anger and sadness switch to that of love then back to anger. Suddenly I recalled one time asking my dedicated nurse mother if she ever saw someone die. "Yes," she replied.

"What do you do when someone dies?" I said with the innocence of a curious child.

"You just accept it and do your job," she stated.

There I was across from my husband looking into his shocked brown eyes that flickered between emotions. I could feel the strong women I am descended from standing behind me and telling me that I needed to accept this moment and go to work because my husband couldn't right now.

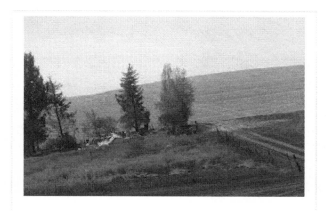

One of the houses that burnt down.

Side-by-side my ancestors, I imagined the Sisters of Providence who founded SHMC and worked and managed the hospital for much of my mother's time there, holding my grandmother's and great-grandmother's hands as they encouraged me to go forth and help my grief-stricken husband.

The next week and the week before the Yale Road Fire my focus became my husband and laying to rest his father who died unexpectedly.

Normally during this time of the year I'm hyperaware about the potential for wildfire. I pay attention to the winds, make a green barrier around my house, and remove flammable debris. This past week though had been spent making funeral plans. This Sunday, Aug. 21 the day after the funeral for my husband's father, was supposed to be a recovery day. Quiet and calm as we found a place for his pets and sank back into our country home before figuring out how to do life with one less person in the world who loved us, we drove home.

Less than an hour later life was anything but calm. I heard the wildfire closing in. It sounded like a combination of the put put of an old engine and the slow banging of a timpani drum. Going vroom vroom, I could hear the fire approaching.

Across the street at my neighbors, quiet became a quagmire as they ran in the house to grab plastic containers of household goods and precious belongings. I yelled across the street, "Are we evacuating?"

"Yes Tammy we are evacuating," someone replied.

I turned around to gather a few things, my daughter and went to get in my car and realized my car wasn't here. We had left our other vehicle at my husband's brother's and my car was now being used by my husband to investigate the fire.

I called his cell phone about 10 times with no answer. Finally I got through, "Get home now! I don't have a car to get out of here!"

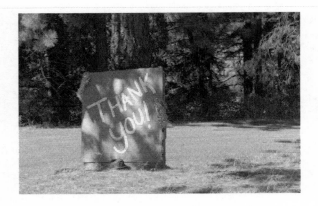

One of many signs created by thankful citizens of Valleyford.

While I waited for him to return I went inside to grab a few clothes and toiletries. On the way out I managed to grab my out-of-print copy of *Warrior of the Mist: A Biography of Qualchan Chief Owhi's Son*. The book tells of the great Yakama warrior Qualchan and his fight against the white settlers and Colonel George Wright in the 19th century. He died in September of 1858 by hanging. This incident took place very close to my home and I grew up next to what is called the Hangman Valley. Being that Qualchan died so near my house has always caused me to have an intense interest with the fallen warrior. It took me months to find this book. I didn't want to lose it. Now the Hangman Valley near Valleyford named after the way he died vs. who he was, currently sprouted flames and made the haunting sound that is wildfire.

My husband returned and we got the dogs and climbed in and took off leaving behind the cats and the chickens.

Now on the road north of the ravine at the bottom of my property I stood jumbling my words while trying to tell someone about the wildfire.

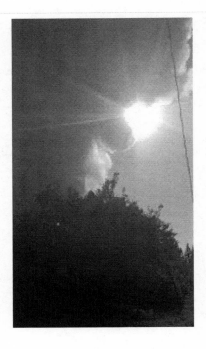

This was what I saw from my house the day the fire started.

My neighbors and I all looked towards our houses now backlit by plumes of smoke. The flames approached and I thought that this was it. My house would soon be rubble. My 5-year-old sat in the back seat and because I hadn't yet figured out how to get the child locks on, kept opening it and saying she wanted to stand near her mama. I kept telling her no and finally walked to the car to keep her from opening the door. I looked ahead at the gravel road that stretched in front of me and saw a large combine coming my direction.

Acclimating to rural life in Valleyford includes navigating around combines. During the parts of the year the combines are out plowing the fields, I plan on an extra 15 minutes into town in case I get stuck behind a tractor.

This time was different. Although still somewhat slow, I could tell this giant farm machine was running at full speed and in a hurry. I yelled at my daughter that she better not open the door. Thankfully she listened as I ducked behind the car just in time to get out of the way of the large metal spirals that went right past my head.

The farmers worked side-by-side the firefighters making plow lines, putting fires out with shovels and axes. Able townspeople went to the many small farms that spot the countryside to help load up horses, pigs and sheep in trailers to evacuate.

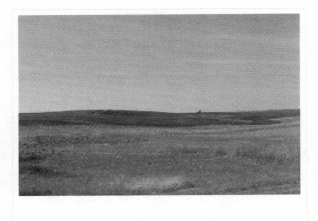

The fire line

Despite saving efforts, many were not so lucky as to get their livestock out. One family lost 400 head of sheep. More than 6,800 acres caught fire in what is now referred to as the Yale Road Fire.

A broken branch colliding with a power line is what sparked the great blaze that consumed much of Rock Canyon and Qualchan's Hangman Valley. The fire started in Spangle and moved so fast it spread quickly into Valleyford and went all the way up to Stoughton Rd. threatening many homes and farms in the area. Ten homes were lost in the fire. It spread so quickly that many didn't have time to get anything out of their house and were left with nothing.

We were Level 3 evacuated twice. Level 3 evacuation means "Get out now!" The second Level 3 evacuation came the next day when the canyon behind my house caught fire. During the second evacuation we managed to get our cat and baby chickens along with our dogs and take them to the fairgrounds where emergency shelter had been set up for animals impacted by the fire.

On the Sunday the fire began, when my husband finally convinced me to leave the ravine facing my house, returning to the vehicle I got in wearing the same face he had been wearing the last week. While nothing can replace the loss of a family member, the fear that I was about to lose my childhood home- the one that my dad spent 40 years of his life building on, welding, caretaking-sank into my soul.

Driving away from the fire that somehow steered away from my home and was now just east, I thought about what it meant to be strong in the face of disaster. I thought about the combines I saw heading into the fire. I looked up at the sky and saw a group of small planes headed toward the flames. We came up with the idea to go back to our house and try and get more belongings. Headed down Stoughton, just before the small forest that signaled we were almost home, I witnessed a plane dump fire retardant on a field I normally see on my morning runs as the home of a couple horses that spend most days gnawing on grass and meandering around in. Now the horses were no-where in sight and the field of mostly alfalfa now grew smoke and flames.

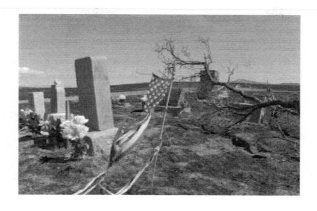

The Valleyford Cemetery after the fire.

My husband turned us around and dropped us off at the Valleyford Church, said he was headed back and pulled out of the driveway. Standing at the church with a group of stunned onlookers the large 747 aerial fire fighter planes flew above me in the skies and toward the giant fire. The street of Madison, the main strip, normally quiet now ran like a freeway as trucks with horse trailers and boats attached moved out of the fire zone.

I lived through the Hangman Fire of 1987. I remember the canyon burning. Like the Yale Road Fire, homes were lost. This fire somehow seemed different. Maybe because I wore the innocent goggles of childhood and I was now experiencing wildfire as an adult, I still have never seen a fire come so close to my town. This time I saw what is referred to as a fire tornado. It's as horrible as it sounds. The most evil destructive natural thing I have ever witnessed.

Although strong on the outside, during this time I was very aware that if I didn't watch myself it could very easily be me in the Emergency Room. I have a disease called Cyclic Vomiting Syndrome. There is very little information on this disease, but they do know that stress can trigger an episode. I spent weeks barely sleeping, not watching my diet (except for no wheat or lentils), and not taking my enzymes (Co-Q10, L-Carnitine, Creatine). For me, that's a recipe for an Emergency Room visit. Thankfully I have people in my life who care enough to call. Care enough to call and ask me if I was taking care of myself during this stressful time. I can't thank you enough friends and family. Perhaps you don't know it, but you saved me from the trouble an Emergency Room visit and being knocked off my feet brings.

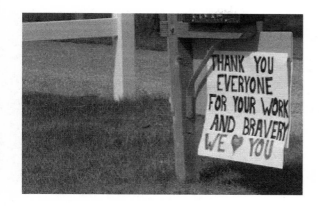

They say what doesn't kill you makes you stronger. I now know that the tough women that came before me are right there standing behind me keeping me strong. I also know that I live in a community that when faced with adversity come together. I told my panicked daughter, traumatized by the possibility that she may lose her home, that we live in a world of helpers and superheroes; many in the shape of firefighters that are here to protect us from the devastation that is wildfire. This quieted her non-stop distraught crying. To my awe, I also now know that in my community, that farmers don't simply work 12-16 hour days to keep us fed. When disaster strikes, they are and were willing to jump into the flames to save all of us from devastation. I know many of the farmers out here are third and fourth generation. I imagine that when this fire struck, the brave farmers-no longer

here but in spirit-stood behind them as they worked to put out the

flames. During this historic fire, we were firefighter strong and

farmer strong.

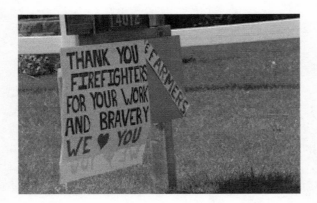

How Strength Brings Out the Best and Worst of People

That saying *What doesn't kill you, makes you stronger* shakes me. I was raised farm, I was raised to be strong. For some people I suppose that saying should read *What doesn't kill you, makes you run.*

That is why when I'm referencing my husband in regards to this book it actually means my ex-husband. It turned out that my father-in-law dying, the Yale Road Fire and other events made him run into the arms of another while I was keeping the fires burning in my own fire house.

For several reasons, I know I have to be very transparent about this. I was married for ten years. I was there for the long haul and stepped up when I had to. I will go to my grave saying he was once a wonderful man whom I was proud to call my husband. He is that no more unfortunately. The last year of our marriage was simply too much for him and he left.

I'm not proud of this for several reasons. One is my religion. I signed a contract and took vows under God. However, he did too. That contract and those vows didn't mean as much to him I guess. I had to let go. I hate letting go. For that reason, I'm not proud that my marriage ended. It did end though.

It ended in a way that I only have God to thank for. I know, divorce is supposed to be an abomination. All I can really answer to that God works in mysterious ways. I ended up being in between a rock and a hard place and God took over and revealed to me things I did not know that were happening in my marriage. In the event that a third person comes into your marriage there is very little you can do to save it. I know this now. I didn't know this then.

It was very hard to let go of my marriage. But I had to let go. Honestly, it came at a wondrous time. I can't say my marriage was pure paradise. It had its ups and downs. Still, I was married. I took vows and I signed a contract. I wanted to fix my marriage. I did not know that the person I was supposed to be working with was working on a new relationship with someone else. Had I known that I would have thrown in the towel then and there.

People ask me the most how this is affecting me knowing that I am chronically ill and have been devastated by divorce. Honestly, this couldn't have come at better time. My illness is virtually abated. I went from considering going on disability – even scheduling an appointment – to having muscles and finding a love for diet and exercise. I have stellar health and prayer. I love my life. I'm sorry that it ended with him, but I have to except that I did everything I did to save my marriage and move on. You can't look back. You must move forward. I get to move forward knowing that I kicked my chronic illness to the curb. I will always be chronically ill, but I have it controlled. That is the most wonderful thing I have ever experienced besides the birth of my child.

I remember the day I realized that wheat might be triggering my vomiting. After 24 hours my entire body changed. I had pain in my stomach that I didn't even know was there. When the pain went away I took a deep breath and fell to my knees. I couldn't believe that I could feel this relief. In the next week pains in my joints and my body went away and my hair even changed. Acne cleared up and everything in my life changed. As things on my body became clearer, things became clearer in my mind. I noticed certain things about my husband I never saw before. I saw how he was able to excuse nearly every nefarious thing he did – including infidelity. For the last year of my marriage he was on the phone commiserating with someone about me. Me, the woman who had birthed his child and stood by him. I even wrote his father's obituary when he died. Suddenly, I was terrible. I was awful. He wanted to leave me.

In the end I let him go. I let him go like I let the pain in my stomach that I had had go that had been there for three decades. Again, I am not glad it ended. I am not glad I am a marriage statistic. I am not glad that I proved how marriage is in trouble these days. I was always taught that marriage was sacred. I still believe this. I believe this even more now. I know what I did wrong. I know what he did wrong. I know why it ended. If I ever have the wonderful opportunity to get married again I know what choices I'll make and what I will do differently.

Life does go on. I have my health. Before I had a marriage and poor health. Now I only have good health. I do have prayer. I did get a wonderful daughter from it. Still, it was a blow. I was betrayed. I do refuse to become bitter. I wish to grow from this. They say what doesn't kill you, makes you stronger. I hope this too will make me stronger. I am so thankful for everything in my life. I am thankful for my mistakes, my marriage and my regrets. Most of all, I am thankful for my daughter and would not change a single thing. She is my gift from God and my reason for

choosing to stay alive. She is my miracle.

That Health Pyramid Thingy

In Maslow's hierarchy of needs it is spelled out in a pyramid what a person needs in order to reach the top of the pyramid. That being the self-actualization. Us humans are innately curious. That's a given, but we wont get the answers until we reach the top of the pyramid.

I'm the first to say that I have a lot going for me in the lower points of the pyramid created by master psychologist Abraham Maslow. At the bottom of the pyramid is the physiological needs of a human. That is sleep, food, water, bathroom. That's what we need to function. Oh, and basic health. I had everything but basic health. Well, I did some of the time. Other times I was very sick with a disorder that was vastly misunderstood and is still mysterious in many ways. But, my basic physiological needs were met as well as they could. I almost always felt safe. I had love and I had belonging. I had pretty good esteem for someone who was sick regularly. There were times I did want the pain from my illness to end. I wanted it to stop. But I never took extreme measures to stop it until I decided to hit the gym.

It was that top part of the pyramid I was never able to reach. That's the self-actualization. I did reach this once I really started to become more healthy. I call it my awakening. Before this I had never had actual dreams. I always made short-term goals. Before this I never even knew what it meant to have dreams for the future. My dreams always consisted of staying out of the Emergency Room for a year. I never achieved this. Now, I take staying out of the hospital for granted – almost. I still thank the heavens every night that I get to experience good health. I also thank God almost every day for not answering my prayers for death when I was sick and in pain on a hospital gurney.

That's where the autistic connection comes into play the most. I've been called Lady Spock my whole life. I always made the most logical choice. I never made the emotional choice. That is because a person cannot be ruled by their gut when their gut is compromised. Really, what is Mr. Spock without Captain Kirk? We need both to really thrive and not just survive.

I feel like when my health came to me a cloud was lifted. That cloud almost caused my life perspective to become translucent not transparent. I feel that I live my life and see things with the full transparency of a piece of cellophane. I began to see how my life choices had been somewhat made in error. That included my marriage. Marriage vows should be uttered honestly with integrity. I thought I did that, but once I started to feel better I thought maybe I had made those promises under the guise of desperation, not honesty. That's a big regret for me.

A regret that I have to live with, mind you. Again, hindsight is 20/20 and I didn't know that I was taking those vows with Swiss cheese health not whole health. I hope you can learn from my mistakes. If you get married, make sure you are holding a full pyramid.

More on the pyramid:

Here's the history as it is some pretty important stuff. So the main guy that came up with it was named Abraham Maslow. It first appeared in a paper he wrote in 1943 called *A Theory of Human Motivation.* This is a big part if developmental psychology. In the process of a developing human, a person goes through many stages before reaching what Maslow calls "Self Transcendant Needs." He studied brilliant humans such as Albert Einstein, Jane Addams, Eleanor Roosevelt and Frederick Douglass to really look at how intelligence goes along with health.

While it was my high I.Q. that ultimately saved me, it wasn't until my health caught up with my brain that I was able to understand spirituality. I was raised a Seventh Day Adventist my entire life. When I had my own child I taught her about Christianity because that was what I had been taught to believe. I fell short a lot in my religion, but it was a wonderful start. However, I didn't truly start having a spiritual relationship until my health was fully in check. It was then that I really pondered what I was doing in my marriage and what I was fighting for. It was then I stopped pouring my energy into it and started putting my energy into my religion.

I have a relationship with Jesus Christ and with God. I do feel it was God who freed me from my marriage. It was his plan that I have to accept. Before my self-actualization I practiced my beliefs, I fell a lot on my journey to wellness and self-actualization. While I practiced living like I was taught, I never truly believed it until I had good health. That begs the question for me on what would someone do if they didn't have the childhood I had. If they aren't at self-actualization they simply don't have the ability to make good decisions. Not being at the top of the pyramid affects evert aspect of learning, thinking and doing. They aren't performing with a full deck. This is an Seventh Day Adventist tenant by-the-way. Seventh Day Adventists do believe that a person has to be at their most healthy and best to find God and/or spirituality. That is why so many of us go into healthcare or social work positions. We are there to heal the body so God can help them decide if they'll let him in their hearts. My heart wasn't truly ready until my body was healed. I healed it because I was able to research good health and make the changes I needed to reach peak performance and health. I learned to Live Better with Chronic Illness.

My Fool-Proof Stay-Out-Of-The-Emergency-Room Diet That

Incidentally Did Not Work BTW

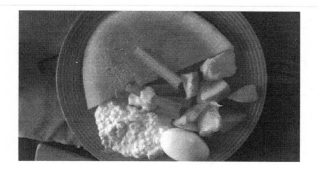

One example of a meal I eat. Cottage cheese, carrots, slice of

watermelon, and sliced peaches. I eat mainly whole foods that

provide simple good nutrition.

My disease Cyclic Vomiting Syndrome took years, no decades

to diagnose.

With Cyclic Vomiting Syndrome, a sufferer experiences extreme bouts of vomiting that last days if not weeks. Usually, a sufferer of CVS will have to go to the Emergency Room to have trained medical personnel help stop the symptoms.

A person with CVS will experience this several times per year. In addition to the necessity of medical intervention, the disease itself is still relatively unknown to nurses and doctors. Plus, the disease often gets misdiagnosed. Before I started going to the Emergency Room my symptoms were always cared for by my mother who is a retired nurse. When my symptoms became so bad, I finally began seeking answers to what I thought were extreme stomach flus or food poisoning.

At first I was misdiagnosed with celiac disease, until finally I saw a gastroenterologist who said I had CVS. Before either diagnosis I thought I had a weak immune system. It seemed logical to me that I live as healthy lifestyle as I could. For sure I was not perfect. I had plenty of indulgences. For the most part though, I ate organic plant-based foods and was mostly vegetarian or I mainly ate fish as my protein source. I read everything I could on what science defined as a healthy diet. I followed it as best I could. For some reason though, my stomach flus got more frequent. I noticed the more foods like lentils and heavy grained wheat bread I ate the more food got vomited into the toilet.

When my daughter was about 6 months old I came down with an episode hours after making a dinner of homemade butternut squash soup and biscuits. Having made everything from scratch, I was able to narrow down what the agitating food might have been, were that the cause of my symptoms the last 30 years. That food happened to be wheat. For the next 24 hours I went off wheat. Almost immediately I noticed changes to my body. Stomach pain I didn't even realize I had abated. For the next week all I ate were steak and M&Ms. My adult acne disappeared, my stomach continued improving, even my hair felt less greasy and more manageable. Not someone who generally follows trends, overnight I became one of those gluten haters.

Months followed no wheat and no sudden CVS symptoms. Still though, occasionally when the norovirus came around I would catch it and my stomach flu sent me to the hospital. I still had cyclical vomiting, although greatly lessened. This continued until my gastroenterologist diagnosed me with a disorder, not a weak immune system. Following a healthy diet, for me, is as easy as pie. Before diagnosis healthy eating was my mantra and I still kept getting sicker. Now I eat a very simple healthy whole foods diet. I eat eggs laid by my chickens with bacon and fruit juice for breakfast. I eat salads without croutons for lunch topped with grilled chicken. I have a small steak with a side of potato and a green vegetable like asparagus for dinner. Milk still bothers my stomach as well as most beans. Wheat is an absolute no. My indulgence: Cheetos. Do I binge. Nope. Do I eat them. Enjoy their crunch. Sure Do. But mainly I focus on eating a well-balanced plant-based diet with about a fist-sized protein per meal like scrambled eggs, chicken breast, or small steak. I also take enzymes that aide in the ATP energy system and the mitochondria like C0-Q10, L-Carnitine, Creatine.

My diet is so simple. Eating healthy isn't a mountain. It's easy. Anyone can do it. It's one of those things that looks difficult, but is really a piece of cake.

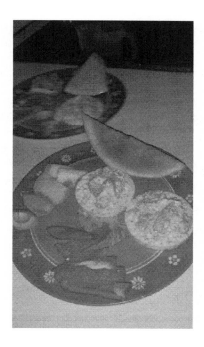

My Gut and My Asperger's

Yes, I'm a little off. I'm kind of weird. Well, walk a mile in my shoes and you may understand. I am a fully functional adult. I take care of business. I just have a really high I.Q. Maybe that's Asperger's, I really don't know.

Take away the gut pain I experienced for three decades, and I'm still a little off. I'm just better at fitting in.

Before, it was always hard to have small talk with people. Think about it though, if you had pain you didn't even know you had would you really be able to have small talk with people. It's not like I was rude, I just didn't engage with others. I didn't have the energy to do so. That's how I learned to survive. I could only really function enough to work and live I was not thriving. I was barely surviving. You can only really thrive if you've reached self-actualization. That's what I learned from living with my illness for three decades.

I was at the gym a year or so back and soaking it up in a hot tub. A man across from me said I was like a beam of light. Yeah, I am happy. I can't begin to tell you what it feels like to be shackled with pain for three decades then feel the joy that is freedom from pain. I actually want to talk to people now. Before, I would close my curtains and sleep away the pain. If I was asleep, I wasn't in pain. Now, I love waking up in the morning. I love seeing the sun rise and the sun set. I am so happy that my journey to wellness led me down this road.

The day I discovered I had a condition and not a weak immune system I felt my physical body change and improve as I changed my workout habits and my diet. As my body changed and improved I became more able to make good decisions and to discover my spirituality. I was awakened. I had an awakening.

Perhaps that was my Asperger's. I was always very smart. I always made very logical decisions. But it wasn't until after I abated the symptoms of my illness that I realized what it meant to be human. I realized what it meant to make decisions of the heart and to make decisions with the brain. There is no Captain Kirk without Mr. Spock and there is no Mr. Spock with Captain Kirk. Together they are what it means to be human. I was a very functional adult. I knew how to function, but I never realized what it meant to be human until after I abated the symptoms of my chronic illness.

I'm afraid this self-actualization has left me with more questions than answers. Although, I get to ask the questions now free from the pain that comes with extreme bouts of vomiting that last for days. I feel for the first time now the pain that is being human. The things that we think about that I was too distracted by my illness to be bothered with. I think those things now. I think them all the time and fully. I am now innately very curious about what it means to be human.

To examine humanity is akin to examining spirituality. What does it mean to be spiritual? I grew up in a religion, but wasn't able to do more than practice it until my health was to par with how a human should feel. Being human hurts. I almost wish I still had stomach pain. Seriously, that was a total exaggeration. Although, being human does hurt.

Probably what hurts the most is knowing that I have to choose to be spiritual. I have to be the one who walks through the door when God opens it. Animals don't have to do this. Humans do. God will open the door, but it is us who has to make the choice to walk through it. That is very hard to do – especially if we have yet to reach self-actualization.

More About My Divorce

As I am writing this, I just finalized my divorce. I'm still examining the choices I made to get married in the first place. I made a huge misstep. I wasn't fully able to have taken those vows, but the buck does stop here. I took them. I made the mistake. Here's a little piece I wrote a few months back that gives a few more details.

Cutting up our fence I stopped. I took a breath. I exhaled. The fog from my exhale wafted in the icy air before it lifted into the sky above me and disappeared into the clouds.

My fence was now in a pile at my feet. I picked up some of the wood and took it inside to my fireplace. Two days into a power outage caused by a windstorm and all I had done the last 48 hours was stoke the fireplace and look for wood.

My husband was nowhere in sight. He had left for work and been gone for two weeks. Although I cared about him deeply, a part of me was beginning to think that perhaps I didn't actually need him. Here I was on my own, building my own fires and cooking my own food. I was able to stoke the fireplace to keep the house warm. I was starting to feel at peace by myself. I felt a sense of strength that I could be- would be okay on my own.

We had been married for eight years and for the longest time, I assumed my life was permanently entangled into his. I never made a decision or had a thought that didn't include him. I had been taught to sacrifice my own needs in the marriage. I defined marriage as compromise. It was something I was willing to do because I married him.

I was 100% dedicated (in every sense of the word) to being his wife - his one and only wife. I took my job as a wife seriously and patterned myself after housewives in the 1950s.

I walked away from a professional writing desk and into a kitchen. A kitchen where I made and served homemade meals on a daily basis and wore an apron. I continued writing short stories and articles for clients and writing fiction for myself. I did this while tending to his every need. He enjoyed every minute of it. If he had ever asked me to stop writing, I probably would have left him then and there. Writing was my outlet – my way of handling the demands of being a full time wife.

I've rearranged words since I was 15. It's as much a part of me as anything. Writing to me is like an appendage. One that cannot be removed.

When I began to suspect he was cheating, something clicked inside me. I felt an intuition that things had changed. I used the skills of research and investigating from my career days. It didn't take me long to find women's belongings around the house. I truly feel this was intentional. He wanted me to find the items to see how I would react. He wanted me to care.

When I would find the things he intentionally left out I would ask him and he just would shrug his shoulders and act like I didn't know what I was talking about. This made me very sad. It was like he didn't even care about my reaction and that my feelings didn't matter.

So, I did what any woman would. I looked in his social media accounts and there it was—a conversation with another woman. The discussion was sexual and how "revolutionized" she was in the bedroom.

I now realize that he left the women's belongings for me to find because he wanted to communicate with me. He wanted me to know what he was doing and to see if I would stop him. In a way, he was trying to "convince" himself that what he was doing was actually okay. I also learned that in a lot of ways he was doing this to hurt and abuse me. He wanted to make me feel pain. He wanted to hurt me.

When I saw the sexual messages, my hands shook at the revelation. At the time I couldn't rationalize the feelings, but it was betrayal. I had given him everything. I'd made him a home. I had sacrificed my career. Now here I was with my landline phone dead, the only connection to the outside world was my cell phone.

I confronted him. He admitted to it. Stupidly I forgave him.

Eventually I worked it out with him, and let him make choices that maybe weren't right for the family, but made him happy. I thought at the time that this is what I was supposed to do. It wasn't. I was blinded by love.

I bent over to make him happy. I even searched for a job outside the home to help with financial concerns. Now that I look back, I did this to try and establish a bit of independence. He didn't really want me to go back to work. Miraculously I never found a job outside the home and for this I'm so thankful. Instead, I focused on my writing. I made extra money doing what I have always done—writing.

During the third power-outage night caused by the windstorm that left me without power for a week, blanketed by total dark and my husband gone, I knew I had to deal with being alone in the dark. It was the only way to keep him from yet again straying.

The only way to make him happy. I thought the reason he cheated me was that there was something wrong with me – that I was too dependent on him.

Still, I got through the major power outage on my own and even learned a new way to cook food over the fire. I even learned how to build my own fire. This made me proud and proved that I was stronger than I thought.

A few more months past after the storm and for some reason I developed this pretty serious fear of driving. It got so bad, I would go out of my way to not take any left turns. Terrified my car would cease in the middle of the road and I would be stuck and everyone around me would have their commute ruined.

I know now, that my driving anxiety was actually my reaction to there not being something right in my relationship. He was cheating. Maybe love blinded my eyes, but it didn't my body. This was my mind and body's way of telling me that something wasn't right.

And it was right. Although we had worked things out, I still felt like something wasn't right. So, when my husband came back from another business trip, I just had to check things out. I checked his phone and apparently he had gone to a town to see his lover. He went where she lived. Through his phone, I could see that he had created a fake social media account to talk to her.

I went into the bathroom and cried. I called my best friend. I went on a run. I ran down the road and yelled aloud, "This will not destroy my soul! I will recover."

That's when I began physically separating from him. I started to work again and make my own money. I literally threw myself into my work. I was already separated from him emotionally. I knew from the black-out that I could make it on my own.

I started visiting friends without him. Although I still had a life with him. I reclaimed my life without him. Yes, we were still married and I knew that divorces took time. Still, I wasn't going to waste anymore time being miserable. He was cheating, and I was done.

When it was time to actually file for divorce, I got a call. It was him. His father was in the cardiac intensive care unit. Later that evening, his father died. I didn't file the divorce papers. I wrote his father's obituary and planned his dad's funeral. I did what any wife would do. I couldn't leave him right then. I wasn't that type of cold-hearted person.

Later after the funeral I looked again at his phone. It had a text on there from this time a different woman. This was a woman he had met only months after the second time I caught him cheating. The text read, "I can come over if you don't want to be alone."

I simply could not understand this text. This was a different woman. A lady I had met. She knew me. She knew he wasn't alone. I pondered the extent of their relationship and what he had even told her about me. Again, I had a feeling that there was something more to their relationship but, I tried to block it out of my mind. I continued to put his needs first. I helped him get his father's belongings into storage and deal with this horrible loss which he had just experienced.

Recently, he left me for this new other woman. The first month I experienced joy. I rekindled friendships. I felt the happiest I had ever felt. I did not realize how much this man brought me down. Moreover, I didn't realize how much all his lies and cheating affected me. I was coming apart at the seams. My driving anxiety, which I was about to go to a therapist for, had ceased.

Moreover, I am daily finding myself in the process of healing for the way he treated me. Everyday I feel lighter and happier. I smile more. By the end of the marriage, I felt such misery. I stopped trusting myself. I lived in fear that he would do it over and over again. He is a serial cheater.

Perhaps the strangest thing about him leaving, is how others have responded. They want to know if I want to talk. At first I thought, "I'm the happiest I have ever been. Why would I need to talk?" But, in all honesty, sometimes I feel pure loneliness.

Sometimes I think about how much I loved him. Sometimes I think of loving someone else. Sometimes I wonder if I'll be alone – forever.

Staying with my ex-husband after the first time I discovered him cheating was my mistake. I didn't fully grasp what being cheated on would do to me. I didn't realize how much it would crush and change me as a person. Over and over again, I wanted to be the good wife – the bigger person. I give him chance after chance. I wanted us to work things out.

The thing was, his problem wasn't us, it was that he didn't appreciate me. He didn't respect me or himself. He was incapable of true love. He took me for granted and I allowed him.

Currently, I feel sorry for him. His new relationship is not working out. I will not be taking him back. The end had gotten so bad, there is no feasible way I will ever get back with him. Plus, I am lonely, but not lonely enough to want to ever be with him again.

Life Lesson:

Probably what I have learned the most from this experience is that when someone cheats on you it's time to end it. He or she will likely just do it again. I wasted another two years trying to fix something that was permanently broken. The only thing you can fix is you. You can heal *your* broken heart. You have the strength and the power. You can do it!

Traveling While Chronically Ill

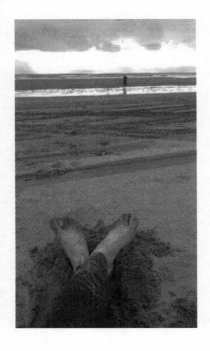

Frequent flyers like me don't travel very far.

That is, frequent flyers of the Emergency Room, like me.

Before I knew I had a chronic incurable disease called Cyclic Vomiting Syndrome, I lived in a pretty scary world.

I always wanted to travel the world, you see, but I was too scared to go very far away from the Emergency Room I was used to.

My disease is one of the most confusing and rare diseases of today, and is often misdiagnosed. If you're into *Grey's Anatomy*, Season 9 Episode 6's subplot is all about cyclical vomiting.

Spoiler Alert!
At the end of the episode, the doctors prescribe the patient Sumatriptan and the patient goes on his merry way having been treated, finally, for his illness. He leaves the Emergency Room with his life improved. But that's not really the story.

The story is how this man was labeled as a drug seeker, then finally the doctors realized the patient had a real illness they had barely heard of. If you're curious about CVS or have CVS and feel alone, this is a good episode to watch.

But this chapter isn't about what CVS sufferers go through in the Emergency Room, that's another chapter. This one's about traveling with chronic illness, or not traveling that is.

Probably one of the strangest things about this disease is that it comes and goes. It has been linked with menstruation and/or stress and has been called the Event Stopper. Reason being, is that this illness pops up around the same time as joyful events, knocks a person out, and they're then labeled flaky and unreliable. With me, I've always worked extra hard at whatever jobs I've had at the time, then when I've become symptomatic and been out sick for a week, it wasn't too much of a stressor for whomever my boss was at the time. I still felt terrible for missing so much work, but now I know it wasn't really my fault.

That's why I've only taken vacations fairly close to home. On one side, I'm worried I'll get sick before I leave and have to cancel my trip; on the other side, I'm worried I'll get sick during my trip and land in the Emergency Room. That's a lot of needless worry for a vacation.

Two nights before we left for the coast I spent the night in a fetal position crying. I kept falling asleep then waking up in the midst of a panic attack that I was about to become symptomatic. Thankfully, because of the enzymes I use and the exercise, I didn't become symptomatic, however.

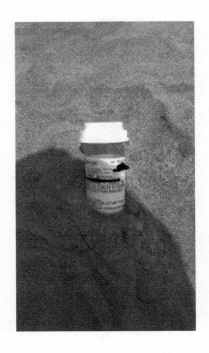

Can't go on a road trip without some emergency
dissolvable Zofran ;)

Because of how I've managed to abate most of my symptoms

through diet and exercise, I didn't do what I normally do on

vacation. I didn't spend the entire time clenched like a fist about

to throw an air punch. I didn't try to do as much as I can the first

day because of the gnawing fear that I may become symptomatic

during my vacation and have to go home early. I had what others

take for granted. I had a normal happy vacation. I ate steamed

clams, built a sand castle, flew a kite. I was humbled by the

vastness of the ocean as I stood in front of it so small and insignificant. One thing chronic illness has taught me: is to never give up. One thing abating my symptoms has taught me: never take a healthy minute for granted.

I'm a frequent flyer of the Emergency Room. One day, if things keep progressing better, I'll be a frequent flyer of the skies. I know I better start flying though, before I sink back into the abyss that awaits us all.

Why I Left My Home Emergency Room

I love the world I live in. I love my town. I love my dirt. I love my Emergency Room. When I first started going to the Emergency Room, I remember vomiting into a cup they handed me at the check in. I then sat in a chair shoulder-to-shoulder with a stranger with a tissue sticking out of her nose and waited until a hospital bed opened. Sure, the setting wasn't exactly ideal but to me it was home. The thing is that if you were a frequent flyer like I was, your body isn't very predictable. Like a building being torn down, at any given time my body can fail me. I've simply learned to live with this fact. When things about your health aren't stable, you look for stability around you. For me, that was my Emergency Room. It was familiar. When I couldn't control the stability of my body, I at least had the stability of going to the same hospital and seeing some familiar faces. I couldn't control that my body was becoming debilitated as my potassium levels grew less, but I could control what setting this was happening in.

Now, there's so much information out there about this disease. I am confident that now I can go into any Emergency Room and tell them of my diagnosis and I will be treated. Most of my treatments involve anti-allergen meds, Intravenous Zofran and lots of dripping saline to rehydrate me. That's a pretty common treatment for my condition, and I am confident that now that there's so much information about my illness that I will be treated.

That's a big part of why I moved. I did live in the country, and I do want to be closer to the hospital and grocery stores packed with the foods that I eat that are close by. That is the pretty awesome thing about moving. Oh, and body cleansing products. I like those. Here's why.

One time after spending three days hospitalized, the nurse on duty kept telling me to get out of bed and take a shower. It took a lot of prodding from her, but I did that When I got back into my hospital bed she came in. She looked at me with widened eyes and stated, "Wow, you're actually okay looking."

Hooked up to my Iv. Bag I kind of just shrugged and looked at her. I then wondered what I looked like before I took a shower. I've heard that my face gets a red and my eyes swell. My hair gets disheveled and greasy. Basically, I looked like hell. She probably saw me at my very worst.

It's weird how things really can change in a blink of an eye. A few years ago I was a struggling stay-at-home wife and mother. I took my job seriously. I took being a mom as a very serious job. I was diagnosed and then went to the books to maybe figure out a way I could stay here so I could take care of my child that I put on this planet before I knew I was chronically ill.

Now I'm chronically ill and divorced. I'm also a single mother struggling to pay bills the only way I know how: writing. It's weird how fast things change. While I'm chronically ill and my body is compromised, I'm soaring in happiness and health. I feel the vitality my body now exudes. I live a healthy life and I'm very happy – even though it is pretty likely I will not get to find someone to share that happiness with.

I Will Survive Until I Survive No More

Basically, I've survived a lot. I've broken my neck. I've lived through wild fire. I've survived this strange disease. It seems that may be the only thing I'm really good at besides writing. In the grand scheme of things surviving is a really good skill I suppose.

Maybe I am chronically ill, but I put some heat on the pavement with my running now. My daughter has shown no signs of having this weird disease. I feel healthier every day. I don't even regret procreating anymore. There's something about becoming a parent. In no way did I ever want to have a child who had to experience the things I have. This is my journey and you can't protect your children from everything, but that didn't mean I wasn't going to try.

When I broke my neck, shortly after they also told me it was likely I wouldn't be able to have children because of my anatomy. Well, I got pregnant the first time I tried. I knew there was something wrong with me. I didn't know it was a chronic disease, but I thought maybe I could help my daughter by practicing good nutrition. At my desk at my newspaper job, I use to have lined up fruits and veggies and I used to munch on them all day. I didn't know if that would help my daughter growing in my belly, but I wanted to at least try. I wanted her to have the very best. I'm a farm girl at heart. I grew up with a huge garden. As my daughter grew in my belly I thought of myself as the soil. I wanted to have a very nutrient rich soil in order for her to grow and develop healthily. I would only ingest the healthiest foods in order to accomplish that. I changed my diet from fast food to whole foods that included grass-fed beef. I was eating healthy for two.

It was a shock that I was even pregnant. I was going to do everything I could to make her as healthy as I could. She's now six and doesn't have a trace of my illness. I wont know if she escaped the vomit monster until she is grown, but I feel better knowing she is maybe going to be spared my pain. That's what really matters. I survive for her. I survive and thrive for her. I really hope that she is spared my aches and pains. I hope she is spared my mitochondrial issues. I practice good health and nutrition and try and teach it to her. I can only hope that if she

does come down with cyclical vomiting, that there is a cure by

then.

That's Not Just the Creatine, I Sometimes Punch Walls

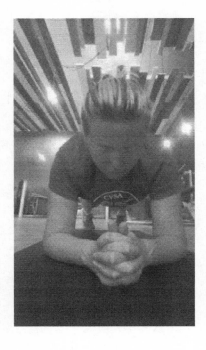

There's a poster on the wall of my gym that asks the question,

"What is your why?"

I'm a book nerd. I don't visualize myself as someone with a

perfect physique who models figure. My "Why" is my daughter.

I knew there was something wrong with me before I had a baby.

If I knew what I know now, I wouldn't have even had a baby. But having a baby is what saved me.

Before procreating, I usually visited the Emergency Room about every three to four months. For years I carried my Emergency Room visits under a cloud of shame. I was ashamed that I was somehow an unhealthy burden to loved ones and medical personnel who were always baffled by my condition. I was often accused of being a drug seeker--even though the first thing they would do was take my blood.

I've noticed, or shall I say my husband noticed, that when I'm taking my creatine I'm a bit aggressive. Because I'm kind of on my own when it comes to treating my disorder, while the enzymes I take are listed as prescribed on my medical chart, I make up my own dosage. In addition to a healthy diet and exercise regime, I take Co-Q10, L-Carnitine, and creatine. Creatine is that powder that body builders use.

My disease, Cyclical Vomiting Syndrome, is currently being studied. Scientists have linked this syndrome with dysfunctional mitochondria. The enzymes I take are all associated with the ATP energy cycle. The mitochondria are the nucleus of every cell in the body but the red blood cells. Therefore, I take these enzymes to increase the effectiveness of my mitochondria. So far I've had a lot of success with my system. I went from being a frequent visitor of the Emergency Room to only going there once in the last three years. I'm not cured, but my life is waaayyyy better.

Before I became pregnant, I knew that morning sickness would probably be pretty epic for me. My obstetrician told me once that I had the worst Hyperemisis Gravidarum he'd ever seen. He'd already been in obstetrics 30 years before meeting me. Go big or go home, I guess. If you're wondering what hyperemis gravidarum is, Princess Kate made it famous with her first pregnancy.

My visits to the emergency room increased exponentially the first months of pregnancy. They were so frequent they finally had to put in a PICC line to keep me hydrated.

Although my visits increased, I was no longer treated like a drug seeker. I was no longer some baffling non-treatable patient. I was now a pregnant woman with a known condition, be it a particularly severe case. Go big or go home.

Not only did having a baby change the way I was treated during my frequent visits, it changed how I treated myself and in many ways caused me to finally get a diagnoses.

When my daughter was 6-months-old I came down with an episode. The idea of caring for an infant while vomiting six times per hour for at least a day, was something that I simply couldn't handle. Thankfully I had some dis-solvable zofran on hand that worked this time. I was safe, for now. A few hours later I examined for the first time what may have triggered this episode.

I hadn't been exposed to the stomach flu, all I had eaten was homemade butternut squash soup I made from scratch. I couldn't be allergic to onions, butter, or squash. I ate those things all the time. The only thing different about my diet was the homemade biscuits I made with the soup. Could it be wheat that was causing this?

I took out wheat and after one day stomach pain I didn't even know I had abated. A week later all my adult acne disappeared. A week later my joint pain went away. I finally understood that I had some sort of condition, I wasn't just prone to the stomach flu. Years later and finally a diagnoses from a gastroenterologist, I'm no longer a frequent visitor and for the first time I'm finding joy in life. All of this wasn't because of me. This all happened because of my daughter.

Not only is she my hero, she is my "Why." I put her on this Earth and she saved MY life. But, it's not supposed to be this way.

She's supposed to be my step into the future, not my saving grace.

Now age five, my daughter tells everyone how her mommy goes to the gym to get strong. She regularly asks if she can work out with me and get strong too. In her mind she sees a mommy dedicated to self improvement. Something I've heard is good for kids. She used to be my buddy in the Emergency Room (no one to watch her on short notice). She was always amazed by my blood draws and how you could make balloons with latex gloves. She has yet to put my gym life and my emergency room life together.

I'm at peace with my body being compromised. I understand that my body is simply not as good nor strong as a normal person's body. I'm not a peace with how I put someone here, and didn't realize this before I did that. My greatest fear is that I put someone here that will soon be abandoned because stupid me didn't realize I wasn't healthy enough to have kids. I often wonder

if and when she'll realize my epic workouts are to keep me out of

the Emergency Room.

When my daughter says she wants to become strong like me

and work out, I want to punch a freakin' wall. Instead of punching

though, I concentrate. Concentrate on staying so I can be there

in case she's the one who needs saving. Maybe it is the creatine

talking when I take it post workout. Users say that side effects

include increased anger. More likely though, it's the gnawing fear

that I won't be here when she really needs me. Every day I'm

getting stronger. It's doubtful though I'll ever get strong enough to

actually make a hole when punching walls. And that's OK. As

long as I'm here.

How Cyclical Vomiting Made Me An Introvert

In my most recent visit to the Emergency Room, my attending physician was at first only slightly interested in my predicament-- which happened to be that I had begun vomiting 8 hours earlier and had yet to stop the recurrent episodes of intense vomiting that had been occurring every 15 minutes since then. He inquired about my condition, then asked if I had used any street drugs or if I was a regular user of marijuana. I told him I did not use marijuana nor any other drug. I then said that I had Cyclic Vomiting Syndrome and I used to be a frequent flyer. However, because of my crazy MacGyver wits, I have abated most of my symptoms.

Laying on my back in the emergency room with an IV. tube sticking out of my arm, I realized how idiotic I sounded at that moment. So I added, "Well, most of my symptoms. I am here."

The doctor reacted at my statement in a way that I had never seen. Most people (I assume) aren't having exactly a good day when they are at the Emergency Room, but for me, my frequent visits were always pretty soul sucking.

I've been belittled by nurses. "People don't have your symptoms! They just don't!"

I've been treated by doctors like I was just another drug seeker. I've been told I either had to get out or get hospitalized, so I've left the Emergency Room while completely high on a cocktail of intravenous Benadryle, Zofran, and whatever else they happened to put in me. During this one visit I remember I was pretty delirious. When they finally got me to leave, I remember having to use the wall in the long hallway from the Emergency Room to my car to keep me from falling. When I did manage to get to my car, it took me about a minute of attempted concentration before I realized I was too doped up on hospital meds to drive, crawled in my back seat, and slept. It. Off.

A lot has changed about the Emergency Room in the three years since they used to treat me then sweep me. For starters, the last time I was there I went straight into a small room and was seen by a nurse who hooked me up with intranvenous fluids and a dose of Zofran before I had even been seen by a doctor. Secondly, my condition now had a name and was known by everyone working in the hospital that day. Thirdly, my attending physician reacted very interested in my syndrome and for the first time wasn't looking at me like I was a giant unfixable inconvenience and just some frequent flyer who needed to be "Treated and Swept off the Emergency Room floor."

He wanted to know how I had stayed away for so long. Cyclic Vomiting Syndrome is barely treatable and incurable. I told him about my diet. I told him about my nutrition and enzymes. I told him about the exercise. His biggest reaction was my elimination of wheat from my diet, "How do you not eat wheat? It's in everything!"

"It keeps me out of here," I replied. "Well, most of the time anyway."

For some reason, humans don't seem to recognize or acknowledge something that they don't understand or doesn't have a name. For years I just had symptoms. Symptoms that were nearly untreatable and so strange that MPs didn't even know how to treat me. Now, my symptoms have greatly lessened, my condition has a name, and doctors and nurses treat me like any other patient. Heaven on Earth!

Being belittled at by medical professionals and kicked out while even more vulnerable when I walked in, wasn't even the worst part. When a person is in the throes of dehydration and compulsive vomiting and finally gets plugged into fluids and the vomiting doesn't cease what do you think is the next logical occurrence? If you guessed that I totally would pee my pants in front of a room full of complete strangers, you guessed right. I have a drawer dedicated to sweat pants that have been gifted to me by the staff of the Emergency Room. Well, I can't say gifted. Most pairs generally costed between $1000 and $5000. Chronic illness is nothing if not expensive.

If you find any humor in my misery let me inform you, my medical chart clearly states, "Patient Has a Sense of Humor."

For some reason uncontrollable vomiting is not exactly pretty. Adults (as far as I'm aware) don't normally pee their pants. There was even an instance where someone asked me point blank, "What the hell is wrong with you?"

"I think I may have been either Hitler or Stalin in a past life. Karma really has a way of showing up, doesn't it?" As my pants became soaked and my emesis bucket runneth over.

Because my illness is defined as an Invisible Illness, after an episode my life would pretty quickly return to normal. Quite possibly, however, my interactions with non-ill humans has caused me to be more introverted than even peeing my pants in front of at least five strangers. I've given up and even lost friends when I've happened to call the day after an episode to check in and see how someone is doing. Here's an example of several phone calls I've had with people after an episode. This is a generalization, but it's a pretty acurate one.

Me: "Hi (so-and-so) this is Tammy."

Them: "What the hell?"

Me: "Suh, huh? I've been sick."

Them: "I haven't heard from you in a week!"

Me: "Yeah I had this weird stomach flu I get all the time. I feel a lot better now."

Them: "I thought we were friends."

Me: "Umm...we are? Or were?"

Them: "I'm not talking to you anymore. People don't get sick like that."

Click or silence.

I've been told that humans do stuff like this to feel more secure in a friendship and I was supposed to call them back and try and work things out. But I didn't. I get now that I'm a bit of an A-hole for not reaching out or calling back. The thing is though, I'm chronically ill. I don't know how many healthy days I have left here. I simply don't have time for that stuff. Dogs don't do that. I think anyway.

I've been told I'm extremely guarded. My question is, "If you walked a day in my shoes, had my experiences, wouldn't you be?"

I'm not guarded. I'm compromised. I'm chronically ill.

On Disordered Eating

I'd like to see the American who hasn't somehow been affected by disordered eating. According to the Diagnostic and Statistical Manual of Mental Disorders, AKA DSM, disordered eating is defined as, "a wide range of irregular eating behaviors that do not warrant a diagnosis of a specific eating disorder."

A specific eating disorder would be something like anorexia or bulimia where the afflicted (generally a female) becomes so obsessed with their body image they forgo the intended purpose of eating (nutrition) in favor of becoming thin. Of course that's just a short definition. There's many layers to either anorexia or overeating. I've seen both the gleam of joy in an overeater's eyes when they indulge in a guilty pleasure and I've been the person pleading with an anorexic to eat so they'll finally lactate and be able to feed their baby.

Seeing disordered eating has been so common in my life, that I was always the odd one who didn't have a weight problem, who didn't overeat (or undereat).

But the nutrition I gave myself was neither normal nor particularly healthy. I went weeks before coming down with a cyclical vomiting episode eating very little. When I recovered I usually binged on food because I had lost so much weight during the episode. After I was diagnosed and began learning about my illness and how to take care of myself I stopped losing 20 lbs every 4 months or so. My body seriously didn't know what to do with itself. On top of that I stopped feeling hungry. On top of that, my body that had been so disordered from my illness that it hung on to every calorie I did manage to consume. So what did I do? I started freak workouts at the gym. It wasn't until I began working out insanely that I could eat like a normal person. Exercise seemed to do more for my body though than make me hungry. I noticed that I felt better than I had ever in my previous life. For the first time I experienced joy in an activity. Anything I ever did before my diagnoses I always had in the back of my mind that I might do something to cause an episode. There is very little out there for people afflicted with this strange illness. I am studying the health sciences in an attempt to heal my body and prevent others from going through what I did.

In the nutrition class that I recently took, the mitochondria was referenced. Through my own research of this illness, I have learned that many scientists attribute dysfunctional mitochondria as being the root cause of this disease. The mitochondria are the nucleus of every cell but the red blood cells. I explain the mitochondria of being like a car battery and our body the car. The car can't start if it has a dead battery. I also found out that aerobic exercise has been found to increase the amount of mitochondria in the muscles as well as increase the effectiveness of it. I'm not a scientist, I'm a journalist. I can't prove with my body's improvement that cyclical vomiting syndrome is caused by defective mitochondria. All I know right now is that I feel wonderful.

When it comes to disordered eating, I feel like my CVS protected me from becoming disordered in eating. Sure, I've had my battles with food. Specifically I was very upset as eating as healthy as I had the last decade only to find out it was healthy foods like wheat and legumes that were actually contributing to my illness.

I eat a balanced diet. It's just nutrition. For people who are disordered because of trauma or because they associate eating with feelings of joy or forbidden pleasure, know that I feel your pain. Although, I never have associated food with anything positive, I've thought of it so negatively that I understand disordered eating. I had to come to terms that I needed to eat to live. So, I understand. I get you.

All In A Name

Onee of William Shakespeare's most frequently uttered quotes, "A rose by any other name would sound as sweet," spoken by the love-struck Juliette in reference to her beau Romeo and his unfortunate last name, makes me think of the name of my own disease Cyclic Vomiting Syndrome. After my diagnoses four years ago this August, I accepted that people would have to know (and picture) that I puke a lot.

I'm not particularly keen on people visualizing me during an episode. And visualize me puking my brains out is something I'm pretty sure happens.

When I worked at summer camps I received quite possibly the best advice when it came to taking care of kids. Don't ever say don't. The reason you don't, is that whenever you say don't, that puts into the recipient of the don't the idea to "do." Still confused? OK. Don't picture pink fluffy elephants. See, you just pictured a pink elephant.

Therefore, when I inform people I have cyclic vomiting syndrome. I know. I just know. They are visualizing me puke. Imagine if you had a disease called Spinning Explosive Diarrhea. You had to tell everyone that you had epic spells of diarrhea. That would kind of suck, huh?

Perhaps I'm too sensitive. When I was pregnant I didn't even tell anyone until I was eight months along. I couldn't handle people visualizing the biological means that causes someone to get pregnant. Everyone just thought I was getting weirdly fat.

Names. They are important. We are given a name when we are born. We name our pets. We name streams. We name oceans. Everything we as humans see or touch has a name. I spent three decades not really understanding I had a condition that had a name. I thought I was more prone than others at getting the stomach flu. I knew that most people weren't hospitalized for the flu. I knew that most people didn't vomit six times per hour. I knew there was something different about my illness. So I gave my illness a name. I called it The Evil Monkey Flu From Hell. Long name, huh? Still, a little more poetic than Cyclic Vomiting

Syndrome.

For those of us suffering with this illness and suffering with telling people the name of your illness, hang in there. Those of us who regularly work with kids give up saying "don't" for one day and try instead giving them constructive things to do. You might be surprised. Or you might not. Kids are pretty unpredictable-- especially that stubborn rebellious Juliette. I mean, her entire family told her do not date Romeo. Look what she did. And what happened?

Cannabis and I are Not Lovers

I always get a load of feedback when I say anything about marijuana. Cannabis really seems to be as polarizing as abortion, political parties, or child rearing. I came into this writing business with a ready-made resentful jelly person just waiting in the wings for the opportunity to find something to criticize me about. Thus, whenever I write about how I DO NOT use marijuana it somehow turns into me using marijuana. Vice versa, people who are regular users completely dismiss me as a 420 hater. Friends, I am neither. The only opinion I have about cannabis is that it's not some magic cure-all. It comes with its own list of side effects. Plus, people call it a natural wonder without considering that a ton of pesticides are used to grow it, and the pesticide use is still unregulated by the federal government--being its usage is still federally illegal.

Before Washington (my stomping ground) State legalized marijuana's recreational usage in 2012 I was always screened at the beginning of my frequent flyer Emergency Room visits as a drug seeker. Yeah it was kind of a pain to have to go through, but after the initial screening I was always treated for my symptoms despite no medical professional being able to diagnose me. And because I WASN'T a drug seeker. At all. I occasionally drink Cabernet. That's it. My body is too compromised to handle anything else. If you're still trying to find something to bring me down to size, humble me, give me what I deserve then know I'm someone who don't smoke no pot. I'm pretty straight and narrow. And when my straight and narrow gets a little too straight I take a 90 degree turn and follow it straight. And BTW, nothing is more humbling than spending hours in the Emergency Room being asked if you use drugs and being accused of getting punched in the gut all the while vomiting every 15 minutes in front of a staff of medical professionals wondering if you're only in the E.R. to get some drugs.

Anyway, after marijuana was legalized in Washington State, things in the Emergency Room changed. I started getting asked specifically if I used marijuana. Soon after its legalization I was officially diagnosed as having a condition known as cyclic vomiting syndrome. From then on, whenever I visited the E.R. medical staff would confuse my illness with something called cannabis hyperemisis. Because my illness is so rare and still so unknown, medical professionals simply see more patients with the cannabis hyperemisis and patients who have it aren't afraid anymore to say that they are regular users of marijuana. Great for them, great for the MPs treating them, not so good for little ol' me.

Even the article in *High Times* states that ceasing use of marijuana will stop CHS. If you're a regular user of marijuana and are somehow still reading this blog, know this: CHS usually inflicts those that use marijuana daily. One study stated that because marijuana has a half life that builds in the system it stays in the intestines and eventually causes stomach pain and CHS.

If you're still reading MJ users, know that regular use of cannabis has side effects. Painful ones. I wouldn't wish my symptoms on ISIS, and there are ways to prevent this from occurring that does not include giving up the now legal wonder drug.

Drinking lots of fluids and regular exercise has been found to help prevent CHS. If that doesn't work give giving up the MJ a chance. C'Mon. You know you want to try it.

Finally a Diagnosis

I really didn't know what to expect when I finally went to see a gastroenterologist more than four years ago. Because of my symptom history I assumed I had some form of celiac disease. I had already cut out wheat from my diet, and was existing under the idea that I had celiac disease. I live in an agricultural area that predominantly grows wheat and have known ancestral farmers with it. My gastroenterologist said that it was unlikely I had celiac disease, however, and my symptoms seemed more like a rare disease called cyclic vomiting syndrome. The disease is so rare in fact it's frequently listed among the most rare diseases of today.

He then told me there was nothing he could do. There was no test for it, no medicine or treatment. The only thing I could do was try Coenzyme Q10.

I'm not someone who takes vitamins on a regular basis. I have, however, taken vitamins in an attempt to maintain my health--to no avail. See, for years I thought I had a weak immune system that caused me to contract the stomach flu more easily and more severe than others. This time when I took Coenzyme Q10 something was different though. My body felt different.

Since I've been on this vitamin, I've only been symptomatic twice in the last four years. That's huge considering I used to have episodes of severe vomiting at least three times per year.

So how and why does this enzyme work? As a journalist I can't help but be curious and even a tad skeptical about taking a pill and suddenly being cured.

Because of my questions about my health and my illness, I've begun taking classes that may lead to a degree in health in addition to my degree in journalism. My latest class nutrition had a lot to say about this enzyme.

Although there is no cure for cyclic vomiting syndrome, it is being studied. Many scientists are correlating cvs with a dysfunction in the mitochondria. Mitochondria are considered the powerhouse to the cells in the body and are in every cell but the red blood cells.

I compare mitochondria to that of a car battery. When you start a car it needs the energy stored in the battery. If its faulty, unless you have a hill and drive a stick, you can't really start your car. If the battery is a tad tricky you could end up with all sorts of car problems. Long story short: keep your car battery healthy.

My mitochondria that transfer energy to the cells of the body don't work like they should. People with mitochondria dysfunction end up with all sorts of health issues--including gastrointestinal and cyclic vomiting.

So how does CoQ10 factor in?

The enzyme CoQ10 is already made in the body. It is also found in a number of foods--especially organ meats. It works in the ATP energy system that makes our bodies function. The same system that houses the mitochondria i.e. our body's car battery.

One of the medical professionals I see even said that issues with the body's mitochondria is something a lot of people are suffering from without even realizing it.

As for ingesting vitamins, most experts are saying nowadays that a normal healthy person doesn't need supplementation. They also advocate eating a healthy diet as a way to ward of disease and maintain good health.

My body doesn't work quite right. That's why I take Co-Q10, L-Carnitine and Creatine. If and when they find a cure for CVS I'll probably stop supplementing. Right now, that's all I can really do. And it seems to be working.

Charles Darwin and I are Best Buds

I'll begin by saying I would NEVER beat a dead horse. I would rent a big truck and probably donate the carcass to some sort of nearby sanctuary that houses and feeds wild cats like Cat Tales. That said, I'll say again that people and I have never really seen eye-to-eye. I try to not make eye contact with them at all actually.

I could go on a huge tangent on why I don't really understand people, but I have stuff to do today like muck out the chicken coop or something.

I think maybe I just don't get First World Problems. I do, however, understand Charles Darwin who's been dead for more than 130 years. People have talked about Charles Darwin's mysterious illness for decades. Much speculation about what it actually was has included chronic sea sickness and Chagas disease, which he supposedly got from a bug bite on one of his voyages. Although, many reports say that he had neither, he actually had some sort of strange chronic disease.

Charles Darwin spent a good portion of his adult life very ill. His symptoms included extreme nausea and vomiting that would last for days then he would go months without any sign of illness. Those same symptoms are the same as those associated with cyclic vomiting syndrome. I was diagnosed with this disease nearly three years ago.

I have so much pity for him. So much so, that if I had the opportunity to travel back in time it would likely be to tell him he has a disease that can possibly be helped by enzyme therapy and exercise. My question is if that would even help? His scientific achievements were so vast, but medicine was surely not like it is today. Plus, had Darwin not suffered would he have worked so hard?

And that's why I see so much in common with the legend. In his journals he describes the miserable illness that plagued him for days--even months--on end. He even lost a daughter to a strange disease, some say tuberculosis but it's really unknown. Today, his decedents mitochondria is being tested to find out if he had cyclic vomiting syndrome or some sort of mitochondrial dysfunction.

Darwin also describes how because of his illness he grew to expect its return and worked zealously when he was well. If Darwin didn't have that drive, would he have made all of his discoveries and changed the world?

That's where I sit with my illness. Had I not had this mysterious disease for three decades, maybe I wouldn't be who I am today?

But the same goes for why I really don't understand people and their first world complaints. I remember when I first took out my main allergen wheat for one day. A deep pain in my stomach that I was so used to that I didn't even know it was there went away. Shortly after the pain abated I thought, "Oh my gosh this is how a healthy person's stomach feels! This is wonderful! Healthy people have nothing to complain about!"

So that last sentence is incorrect. Health is everything, but its not everything...I guess.

I am at peace with how my young life was plagued by a strange disease. When it comes to people, however, let's just say I'm working on it.

In my twenties I had a very poignant conversation with my fiance, now my husband, now my ex-husband. "You know I can't have kids, right? You know I probably wont live much past 30?" Anyone who has ever been in their mid-twenties probably already knows that 30 sounds really far away and really old. I'm assuming that that's likely the reason he kind of brushed off my commentary about my mysterious ailment.

Now in my mid-30s I'm sometimes astounded that I am still here. More surprised then I was at having a kid and not dying by age

30. Not nearly as shocked as I was shortly after turning 30 that I had an actual disease with a name and not just some vile and awkward thing I had to deal with three times per year. I was diagnosed with cyclical vomiting syndrome more than four years ago. That diagnoses changed my life.

This whole blog is dedicated to my illness, so the fact that a simple diagnoses changed my life is a bit of an understatement. Being diagnosed turned me into a gosh dang superhero!

My Disease and the Elephant in the Room

I've had this disease as long as I've had memory. It became a part of my very existence. It's like I spent my childhood, adolescence and twenties carrying an elephant. For imagery sake, let's say the elephant was an adorable baby during my childhood and nearly full-grown in my twenties. I turned 30 and the elephant jumped off my back and rejoined its herd. How did that leave me? It left me with a rock hard back is what it did.

There is no cure for either cyclical vomiting syndrome or mitochondrial disease. But there are people all over the world who've been diagnosed and now know how to manage their disease. I'm one of those lucky people. The heavy load I've carried my entire life has been lifted.

Because my young life had added difficulty, I simply learned how to do life differently. It's a difference that now fills me with joy and my life habits are so beneficial to me. In short, my illness was a blessing. The many blessings of it are listed below.

1. My Bills Are Always Paid Three Months in Advance

I never knew when I'd end up bedridden or in the hospital. All I ever knew was that it was inevitable. My bills were always paid way in advance. I've always had a savings account to pay for any deductible I may acquire.

2. I Achieved All My Goals

Three years into my diagnoses sans fear that my body will fail me, I still don't understand what dreams are. I never had any. I can say now that my dream has always been to go a year without nearly puking to death. I've done that. My dream came true. That said, I did grow up in a generation that promised hard work would lead to the life of your dreams and that with enough sweat equity I could have anything I wanted. Knowing as an adult that the above teaching is complete b.s., I still heard it repeatedly and it taught me to make goals. I made plenty of them. They were small goals like going here or accomplishing this, ect… and I always reached my goal…right before I landed in the emergency room that is.

3. I Don't Care If People Don't Like Me

If someone isn't treating me how I think I should be treated I walk away from them so fast. I didn't ask to be here. I didn't ask to spend a lot of my childhood in a room reading books because I was so sickly I couldn't keep up with other kids. It's not my fault I didn't get to develop like other people. I have a terroir all my own. I don't do anything to anyone. I help people more than most. Sure, I see the world a bit different. But I wouldn't want it any other way. That said, I'm not proud of how little I understand passive communication. I've lost dozens of friends over this. When this happens I call it Sheldon Coopering. Or when I accidentally Sheldon Coopered someone. One example I would use would be that I've been in situations where someone's said, "Man I'm thirsty." My response will usually be, "Oh that sucks." But if someone says to me, "Hey could you get me a drink of water?" I'll always jump up to get it. I don't understand the cause of this. It seems gender-biased, but I don't really have much insight on whether women are expected to understand passive communication better than men. All I know is I've ticked off a lot of people because I don't speak passive. But I always brush it off. Again, I didn't ask to be here or to try and interpret that stuff. I'd much rather be soaking up the sun anyway.

4. I Don't Waste Time Not Liking People

Although I do have a preference for responsible dog lovers- especially flat-coat owners!- I don't waste a minute disliking someone. Honestly, I don't understand why someone "likes" or "dislikes" a person. My character assertions revolve around if I think the person is a sociopath, a narcissist, or someone who is punitive towards others or animals in anyway. If you're none of those, then we're good. I've had people look right at me and tell me they didn't like me because of the shape of my nose. I've also had people tell me they didn't like me because I reminded them of the cheerleaders they went to high school with. The ones they hated (anyone I went to high school with, lets all share a collective chuckle.) One time I even overheard a person explaining to someone else how they didn't like me. This was the conversation: A) Yeah I really don't like her. B) But why? She seems so nice. A) Yeah, I don't know. I just don't.

Yeah, I totally don't get that stuff. It seems like mental illness to me. It seems pretty common though. For the record I am not Autistic nor do I have Asperger's as far as I know. I actually had a test done. People who are either cannot understand wit. I not only understand wit, it's kinda my life. I'm just some lady with a high I.Q who spent her childhood in a room with books. I'm like Nell but with a high I.Q.

5. I Have A High I.Q.

Again, nothing I asked for. In fact, I've referred to my high I.Q. as "The Curse". If I had been able to choose my childhood it would have been right down the middle, not of such a sickly constitution I ended up a well-read adult who constantly calls out other people's b.s. just by happenstance. Another way I don't keep friends.

6. I Get To Be Simple

I still can't believe I get to feel like other people do. I'm no longer carrying a heavy elephant that makes every day harder. I no longer have to spend every day anxious, not anxious about other people or anything I'm doing, but anxious that my body will trip over itself before I have a chance to reach my goal. Now I get to still be sorta young with a healthy body that most people in their 20s and 30s take for granted. I get to be a vibrant part of my community and my world. I have been given the wisdom of empathy to the suffering of others, yet I'm still young enough to be of help. I'm getting to help others maintain their health and have longevity. I get to be salt-of-the-Earth. For that I am blessed.

Why I Don't Look Forward to Cold Weather With Cyclic Vomiting Syndrome

---

I woke up this morning wondering if I could even "do" today. Four years passed my diagnosis of cyclic vomiting syndrome and now I'm forgetting. I'm always reminding people that although invisible, I am chronically ill. My illness is in fact so odd, that I can be fine for months on end and them bam — I'm out of the healthy world for up to two weeks.

On mornings like today I am painfully reminded that although I pass as someone perfectly healthy, I'm far from it. Perhaps the majestic summers I've lived through are what causes me year after year to forget that I am chronically ill? I've had this disease as long as I've had memory and I do not recall ever being symptomatic in the summer.

The ends of September/beginnings of October I've lived through tell a very different tale. Historically, when the weather starts to turn, my stomach starts to churn. When stomach viruses invade public places (usually when it starts to get cold) I become a germaphobe. I carry hand sanitizer at all times and wipe down everything with sanitizing wipes. Normally this does the trick, but sometimes my efforts do not save me from the norovirus. A person who has only experienced the typical stomach flu probably cannot understand why someone with my illness would be terrified of contracting a little stomach bug. Well, let me say that what might be a little stomach bug to you can very easily turn into a trip to the emergency room for me, where I'll lay for hours in a hospital bed while medical professionals draw my blood, insert an IV and give me a cocktail of medicines that are doing who knows what to my body. What may be a tiny stomach inconvenience to you becomes something that has to be treated by medical professionals for me. If not, I can become so dehydrated, my body's organs begin to fail. Every visit to the emergency room comes with the possibility that if I don't get rehydrated and properly treated, it might end with me leaving in a body bag.

I know scientists are researching the different causes of cyclic vomiting syndrome. I've heard stress can be a trigger, as wells as an unbalanced diet. I do not know why me contracting the norovirus can cause a full-blown abdominal migraine, but I do know that I experienced such a severe case of hyperemesis gravidarum when I was pregnant, doctors had to insert a PICC line. I'm guessing my body is just in the habit of going into a full cyclical vomiting episode (experiencing emesis every 15 minutes for days on end).

Mornings like the one I had today reminded me of this. I woke up nauseated and terrified. The cold outside did not help. I took a warm bath. I ate something. I cried. Nothing helped until eventually the stomach pain passed. Now I'm writing this. When this is submitted I'll go about my day posing as a healthy person, taking care of my house and daughter when she gets home. Likely I'll go buy sanitizer and wipes today in preparation for the cold months to come. This morning was a wake-up call. I'm thankful that's all it was and I didn't end up back in the ER. I will be keeping the wipes and sanitizer out and ready these cold months ahead of us in hopes I can go a full winter without seeing an ER doctor.

Four Tips for Getting Through the School Year With Cyclic Vomiting Syndrome

My illness, cyclic vomiting syndrome (CVS), like many other invisible illnesses, comes and goes. Periods of wellness for me would sometimes last for nearly a year. Because of this, and really wanting to be healthy, diagnosing this disease was lengthy and difficult. Finally, after a diagnosis, I realized that many of the challenges I experienced in school were, if not completely caused by, somehow related to my invisible illness.

A student with cyclic vomiting syndrome may encounter many misunderstandings with his or her peers if this disorder is not properly communicated. Because this illness is invisible, it's difficult for healthy people to understand that an adult or a child might be at a disadvantage because of this disease. I've compiled a list of ways to avoid awkward situations where a classroom peers may try engage with you in conflict because of a misunderstanding or a teacher may mistakenly give you a bad grade because they simply don't understand invisible illnesses.

1. Educate the classroom on this disorder.

If you're the parent of a child with CVS, when you drop off your child for their first day of class, make sure your teacher at least knows the student may have a lot of absences. Someone with CVS doesn't often show up for class when they are sick — especially on the first day. For me, the first day of school was always filled with hope for the year. I wish I realized on the first day of class that the year ahead would likely be filled with unexplained lengthy absences and hours on the weekends trying to play catch-up. They need to know the potential for absences is there so they can prepare and not mislabel you or your child as "flaky" or "unreliable."

2. Know the signs.

Although invisible, CVS still has its own set of symptoms and predictors that help foresee when an episode may begin. A CVS episode means experiencing extreme bouts of vomiting that may last days if not weeks if left untreated. A person about to begin an episode will usually look pale and sweaty right before an episode starts. Additionally, a person with this illness will often begin to act listless and become weaker.

3. Consider working ahead.

Between episodes, a person with CVS might consider studying more and working ahead so that when episodes strike, they'll be prepared.

4. Communicate with the teacher.

I'm pretty positive that many of my past peers and teachers still view me as someone who skipped a lot of class to go to the mall. There's nothing to be done about that label other than move on and educate people on invisible illnesses. This is where my past mistakes can be used to help prevent others from experiencing what I did. Tests will missed. Assignments will be turned in late. Don't do what I did and accept an inferior grade or withdrawal from the class. Get your diagnosis results from your gastroenterologist, make sure your teacher sees it and plan on taking your tests on a make-up day.

CVS has been linked to stress, so just when you think you're ready and about to take the test, bam! CVS is right around the corner and will knock you to the ground. Then you're dealing with CVS and the stress of getting a good grade.

These are some of my tips to avoid a CVS episode:

- CVS is linked to stress. Try to avoid it, but if you can't do that, take a class on meditation or find a physical therapy office that does biofeedback.
- Don't go hungry. Fasting may trigger a CVS episode. Carrying snacks with you to avoid hunger may help.

- Consider dissolvable nausea medication. When I first started being treated for CVS, they were using suppositories. Thankfully, you can now get a prescription for nausea medication that you don't have to swallow and you don't have to…well…you know.

Spinning My Mitochondria Into Midi-Chlorians

Who doesn't want to be a Jedi? In order to become one, you gotta

work with the midi-chlorians. According to Qui-Gon Jinn, midi-

chlorians are intelligent microscopic life that live symbiotically in all

life cells. If the numbers are sufficient in the body, the body's host

may be able to detect the force and learn to use it. Thus you

become a Jedi.

In the fairy tale Rumpelstiltskin, the daughter of a simple miller-of-

grain is sentenced to do the impossible in order to save her life. If

she doesn't complete the impossible task of spinning straw into

gold and simultaneously advance her father's station, she will lose

her own status-or in some versions her life-as the king says he will

cut off her head if she doesn't do as promised. It isn't until she

makes a deal with the devil (an imp that appears out of no where)

that she is able to save her own neck and accomplish what others decided she was capable of.

In the end she outsmarts the imp and manages to advance her station and please everyone who originally expected the impossible of her. This tale isn't unlike the impossible task that life has assigned me. Unlike the miller's daughter, however, science is in my favor.

While the miller's daughter had never spun straw into gold, I have had to deal with health situations in the past that most people would possibly falter under if presented to them. Much like the miller's daughter, however, the reason of my survival is somewhat akin to making a deal with the devil.

The devil I'm referring to lies deep within. I'll always remember the look on the off duty EMT's face when my open eyes shook with life upon his approach. I don't recall opening my eyes. The force of the semi that hit me nearly shook the life out of me. Thankfully it didn't completely, as I recall the moment of lifelessness joined by the reemergence of sight. At the same time my lungs started moving my eyes connected with a man approaching my wrecked vehicle. Noticing someone looking at you with the dread that he might be walking towards a dead body that is you is something I'll never forget. Just like I'll never forget the inquisitive look on my physical therapist's face months later when she stated she had never seen someone work as hard to get better as me. I responded, "It really just ticked me off that I had to deal with this, so I'm gonna eat this traumatic brain injury for breakfast."

Perhaps it's not the devil, maybe it's mere survival. I really don't know. What I do know is, I'm ready to deal.

My disease is considered baffling by most medical professionals. Cyclic vomiting syndrome is also ranked as one of the weirdest diseases of today. In reading the scientific journals, however, I have been able to find out that it has been linked to mitochondria dysfunction. So that's where I'm at. Fix my mitochondria and maybe, just maybe, I'll fix me.

Despite this strange disease having no testing nor a cure, our body's mitochondria can be improved. The results of this are evident simply with me. I went from decades of dealing with regular episodes to nearly eliminating any symptoms of this debilitating disease. I ingest enzymes that are part of the ATP energy system in our body. The powerhouse of the system, the mitochondria, plays a heavy part in maintaining the body's function and the functioning of the ATP system. Aerobic exercise increases the mitochondria in the body as well as increasing the effectiveness of the mitochondria. Hooray for me!

Anaerobic exercise involves short duration, high intensity movement. Some examples include heavy weight training sprinting or jumping. Aerobic exercises are those like spinning, heavy cardio and marathon running. The best way to remember it is anaerobic leaves you out of breath in short duration exercises, while aerobic is of longer duration and utilizes oxygen. I'm already someone who likes to exercise. There's nothing like a week in a hospital bed and three months in a halo to tell you any kind of movement is a gift. While I prefer lifting weights, I've made the move to more cardio exercises like spinning and running because I want to perform more aerobic work to increase my body's mitochondria. Therefore I'm spinning (cycling) like I'm trying to turn my mitochondria into the same stuff that Jedi's use, the midi-chlorians. I'm assuming I'll never get to speak to mitochondria and be able to control objects and thoughts with my mind, but you better believe me when I say that that's my goal. At least for now. See in my case, with my strange disease, it's like I am trying to spin straw into gold.

Why I Sometimes Thank Jerks for Their Comments

Even the most uproarious jerk has experienced this. You're out and about. You're living your life like you do and Bam! some person you don't even know has something to say about your clothes, your appearance, or my personal favorite: how you parent.

I don't have a lot of insight as to why people do this. I'm sure I'm probably guilty of doing this on occasion as well.

It's all in how you take it, I guess.

For me, the comments people say about my appearance, I use as a necessary gauge of my health.

Because I have an invisible illness, most people do not understand why I disappear for long periods of time or don't partake in activities that I feel are going to cost me my health i.e. late night parties, bars, extreme social situations. I've only lost a few friends over this. I much prefer hikes, bike rides, the gym, books, movies, and other online games. I've accepted this. And I do engage in more social activities as my illness improves.

Before diagnosis, I called my extreme debilitating flus my Fiona disease. One of the main characters from the movie *Shrek*, Fiona, is cursed with sometimes being a beautiful princess and the rest of the time a transformation occurs that causes her to be an ugly ogre.

When in the first phase of a cyclic vomiting episode my appearance begins to change. Like I am morphing into some hideous monster, my skin sometimes develops an orange cast to it, acnes and rashes appear all over my body, and my hair no matter how much I wash it appears greasy. People who don't suffer from an invisible illness are simply struck by how different I look. They don't understand. Before diagnosis I would get comments like, "You look tired," or "You look like you're having relationship problems."

I still don't understand that one.

Before I knew what was happening to me this, of course, was a little soul-crushing. I simply felt like I wasn't good enough. Then I would disappear for the next week and quite possibly end up at the Emergency Room.

This continued until my diagnosis. Then things changed. As my body began to heal, my face started to glow. My hair stopped looking so disheveled. No one commented about my appearance looking in anyway less than tolerable.

Pretty good sign my life changes were working, huh?

The real kicker with my illness, however, is it has triggers. One of them is stress. They've linked one cause of CVS episodes to be raised cortisol levels in the body.

Here's from one of my favorite research sites, The National

Institute of Diabetes and Digestive and Kidney Disease:

Specific conditions or events may trigger an episode of cyclic vomiting:

-emotional stress, anxiety, or panic attacks—for example, in children, common triggers of anticipatory anxiety are school exams or events, birthday parties, holidays, family conflicts, or travel infections, such as a sinus infection, a respiratory infection, or the flu

-eating certain foods, such as chocolate or cheese, or additives such as caffeine, nitrites—commonly found in cured meats such as hot dogs—and monosodium glutamate, also called MSG

-hot weather

-menstrual periods

-motion sickness

-overeating, fasting or eating right before bedtime

-physical exhaustion or too much exercise

Because of this, I do not have toxic relationships with people. If you're someone who's reading this wondering why I stopped talking to you after an argument or some sort of discourse please understand that I walk away and shut the door on arguments. I'm big on forgiveness, and the reason I never reached out to you is because reaching out to you might land me into the Emergency Room, and not because you knocked a few teeth out like you may have wanted to. I simply can't do that stuff.

That leads me one lucky experience I had when I broke my neck, wore a halo for three months, and had a couple months of physical therapy. Never thought I'd use lucky and broke my neck in the same sentence.

While doing my exit interview, the physical therapist asked me if I was having trouble sleeping. I answered yes, but not because I was in any pain, because I was having nightly panic attacks. After the interview, she introduced me to a gentleman currently getting his doctorate in something called biofeedback. She set me up with several sessions with him.

In a darkened room, he put these thimble things on my fingers that had wires coming out of them and connecting to a computer in front of me.

For the next several weeks, a few days a week I would sit in front of a computer screen and learn to control my blood pressure.

The tool used was a video game. The sensors placed on my finger tips read my blood pressure. If my blood pressure was too high a floating rock going horizontally across the screen would go up. Too low and it would fall down. My job was to keep the rock floating across the screen. This taught me to control my blood pressure and my stress level.

He explained that my panic attacks stemmed from me slipping to my subconscious right before sleep. At this moment right before slumber, a person can't move their limbs. Sort of awake, sort of asleep, and super paranoid about not being able to move, I panicked. These panic attacks I was experiencing were causing all sorts of imbalances in serotonin and other hormones because of the quick fight or flight response or release of adrenaline.

By learning to control my blood pressure, I was able to maintain my stress level during that vulnerable time when a person falls into slumber and stop my panic attacks.

So how does this help me now?

For the most part, I can control how stressful things affect me. For example: After a vacation to the ocean this summer we broke down still several hours from home. During this experience, I started laughing uncontrollably. My husband (now ex-husband) even commented, "Tammy this is really serious."

"I know, I know. I'll call a tow truck," I said while laughing hysterically.

Let's just say the car breaking down was the least stressful thing that has happened this year. I'm only human and I'll say that the stress of life has begun to affect even successful biofeedback patient me.

Lately I've started getting comments on my appearance like, "You look frazzled," or "You look stressed." Finally yesterday I realized I was having a hard time calming myself down. And I started thinking about the little comments tactless people sometimes say. I realized I wasn't in control anymore. So I reached out. I did some self-care and finally, I calmed down.

Thank goodness for people and their little jerk comments. Without them, I might never see that I'm losing the battle with stress and that my body as a result is about to have an abdominal migraine. They are my gauge to my health. So thank you. But only when the biofeedback stops working.

Before we go, I wanted to do a summary of all the facts I just laid down. My greatest wish is that this helps you on your Journey to Wellness. Everything I've been through I consider a gift from God and my biggest hope is I can now help others learn how to Live Better with Chronic Illness.

I Have Cyclic Vomiting Syndrome

This strange disease is currently being studied. It is linked to mitochondrial dysfunction. I am targeting the healing of my mitochondria in order to cure my disease. I did just that. I went from going to the Emergency Room three times a year for a decade to only going occasionally when I get the stomach flu. Fifty percent of the American population goes to the Emergency Room when they get the flu. That's why I now consider myself cured although I am now diagnosed as chronically ill.

My Hospital Visits

I used to be so ill that I had to give up working. I focused on my daughter and curing myself of this disease. I was very close to going on disability as I wasn't sure if I could work. I now work from home. I recently finalized my divorce and have moved. I am no longer fearful of going to an Emergency Room because of the widespread awareness of this illness. Before awareness of this illness I was always labeled a drug seeker. Now, I am treated at the hospital but rarely go as I have abated the symptoms of my illness with enzyme therapy and exercise therapy.

Exercise

Exercise is now a part of my life. It is how I learned how to Live Better with Chronic Illness. I go to the gym frequently. I also take my dog on long walks and if I have a chance to move I do so. My life is so different now with exercise. I have never felt better. I love my existence. Before I was barely surviving. I am now thriving. I did it with aerobic exercise and the grittiness I learned as a child. I run on the treadmill, do jumping jacks or walk. I love to workout!

The Fat Component

I wonder a lot how the low-fat nineties I grew up in impacted my illness. I know that many vitamins we take require fat to properly absorb into the body. Those are known as fat-soluble vitamins. I take enzymes like CoQ10 and L-Carnitine. Most of the other nutrients I ingest I do so through proper nutrition. I put creatine in my smoothies. I'm no fitness model, but I am healthy. Most importantly, I am happy.

Charles Darwin

He spent his life plagued by a debilitating disease that would come and go. He would experience months symptoms free then would get an outbreak of severe vomiting. That's why many people believe he had cyclical vomiting syndrome. I'll never be known as widely as Charles Darwin, but I do have the same disease and through education I was able to unlock the secrets to curing this illness. Even scientists now think the only way to help this illness is with a healthy lifestyle. That's what I did. I am in no way perfect, but now living healthy is vital to my well-being. I turned my life around and learned how to Live Better with Chronic Illness.

The ATP System

Let me caveat by saying that I worked on a lot of cars in my youth. That is why I use a lot of car analogies to compare our body to that of a vehicle. If the mitochondria is the batter, then the ATP system is the alternator. This car part transfers the energy from the car's battery to start the car. If it is faulty, then it can't charge the car right. That's why we need to change the way we eat. We need to eat more whole foods and be more healthy. It really is up to each one of us to make that decision. However, our health depends on it.

Mitochondria

So, the mitochondria are the car battery and our body's cells the car. The mitochondria must be maintained if we want to avoid reoccurring chronic illness. That is why I targeted the mitochondria. The best way to help the mitochondria is through aerobic exercise and eating fruits and veggies.

Enzymes

I take CoQ10, L-Carnitine and Creatine. These enzymes all work in the ATP energy transfer system and occur naturally. If these enzymes are made in low quantities in the body, then all sorts of things happen to the body. Diseases become more frequent and organs become ill functioning. Most of these enzymes can be found in whole foods and do not have to be taken orally. I take these enzymes in pill form because my body is compromised. Basically, it gives my body an extra charge. It's like when your car has a dead battery and you use another car and some spark plugs to jolt it with some extra power.

My Current Lifestyle

I do everything I can to live healthy. I exercise and eat whole foods. I am human. I have many flaws. I make many mistakes. I still wake up in the morning with the intention to be healthy. Most days I succeed, although some days I fall on my face. Still, it is vital that I try. I take vitamins and eat lots of various fruits and vegetables. I take long walks and use the stair stepper at the gym. I try to focus on aerobic or cardio exercises as they improve the function of the mitochondria. I love being able to take charge of my health. I love growing my own vegetables. I love having my own chickens. I love cooking whole food for my daughter. I am

so thankful for my journey to wellness. I truly learned how to Live

Better with Chronic Illness. I thank God for my health every day.

##

48966442R00100

Made in the USA
Middletown, DE
02 October 2017